SILENT MYOCARDIAL ISCHEMIA AND INFARCTION

BASIC AND CLINICAL CARDIOLOGY

Series Editors

Henri Denolin, M.D.
Director of Cardiological Research Center
Hôpital Universitaire Saint-Pierre
Brussels, Belgium

H. J. C. Swan, M.D., Ph.D.
Director, Department of Cardiology
Cedars-Sinai Medical Center
Los Angeles, California

Other Volumes in Preparation

SILENT MYOCARDIAL ISCHEMIA AND INFARCTION

PETER F. COHN

Professor of Medicine
and
Chief, Cardiology Division
State University of New York
Health Sciences Center at Stony Brook
Stony Brook, New York

MARCEL DEKKER, INC.   New York and Basel

Library of Congress Cataloging-in-Publication Data

Cohn, Peter F., [date]
⌐ Silent myocardial ischemia and infarction.

(Basic and clinical cardiology ; v. 5)
Includes bibliographies and index.
1. Coronary heart disease.   2. Heart--Infarction.
I. Title.   II. Series: Basic and clinical cardiology ; 5.
[DNLM: 1. Coronary Disease.   2. Myocardial Infarction.
W1 BA813ST v.5 / WG 300 C6785s]
RC685.C6C586 1985   616.1'23   85-25260
ISBN 0-8247-7469-8

MARCEL DEKKER, INC.
270 Madison Avenue, New York, New York 10016

Current printing (last digit):
10 9 8 7 6 5 4 3 2 1

PRINTED IN THE UNITED STATES OF AMERICA

For
my wife, Joan,
and
my sons, Alan and Clifford

Series Introduction

The series *Basic and Clinical Cardiology* has, as one of its objectives, the presentation of current knowledge on topics of recently recognized importance. "Silent" myocardial ischemia has recently been recognized as an important phenomenon within the broader topic of ischemic heart disease. Although many cardiologists believed that the symptom of angina pectoris was merely the tip of the iceberg, and that electrocardiographic and perhaps mechanical disorders of ventricular function preceded this symptom, the ramifications of these concepts were poorly understood. This volume reflects largely the opinions of a single authority in this important field. Concepts of coronary vasomotion and high-quality dynamic electrocardiography are serving to identify the potential and actual prevalence of such disorders. However, the significance and management implications have yet to be defined. In this regard, Dr. Cohn's monograph is a summary of knowledge on the topic at the present point in time. It also clearly defines major issues to be elucidated in the future. It provides practicing cardiologists with a reference to the direction of this important topic for the future.

H. J. C. Swan

Preface

The purpose of this monograph is to discuss what is known — and what is not known — about asymptomatic coronary artery disease and its two major components: silent myocardial ischemia and silent myocardial infarction. These disorders afflict millions of persons, yet little is written about their mechanisms, prognosis, and other characteristics mainly because physicians — and the lay public — traditionally associate myocardial ischemia and infarction with chest pain (or its equivalents). That this is not necessarily so is becoming more and more evident. Symptomatic episodes may represent only the tip of the iceberg of myocardial ischemia.

To evaluate the subject in a systematic way, this book has been organized into five major parts: pathophysiology, prevalence, detection, prognosis, and management of asymptomatic coronary artery disease.

Many of the studies discussed in the following chapters were performed with the assistance of my colleagues at Harvard Medical School and the Brigham and Women's Hospital in Boston, and the State University of New York Health Sciences Center at Stony Brook. Their contributions are greatly appreciated, as is the expert secretarial assistance of Mrs. Marlene Landesman.

Peter F. Cohn

Contents

SILENT MYOCARDIAL ISCHEMIA AND INFARCTION

Introduction

The realization that not all coronary artery disease must be symptomatic is not a new one, but it has not always received the attention it deserved.

The history of asymptomatic coronary artery disease is basically a history of its two major syndromes — silent myocardial ischemia and silent myocardial infarction. *Silent (painless, asymptomatic) myocardial ischemia* is best defined as objective evidence of transient ischemia (on ECG, radionuclide studies, etc.) in the absence of angina or its usual equivalents. *Silent (unrecognized) myocardial infarction* is essentially an ECG diagnosis. Autopsy reports of extensive coronary disease in persons apparently free of symptoms were the first important clues to the existence of this syndrome [1]. The next important — although indirect — mile-

Table 1   Types of Cases in Which Silent Myocardial Ischemia May
Be Found

I.	In persons who are totally asymptomatic
II.	In persons who are asymptomatic following a myocardial infarction, but still demonstrate active ischemia
III.	In persons with angina who are asymptomatic with some episodes of myocardial ischemia, but not others

stones were studies of unexpected sudden death in which large
numbers of previously asymptomatic persons were involved. But
it was not until patients with coronary artery disease were actually
observed to be free of pain during episodes of transient myocardial
ischemia on exercise tests [2, 3] and during ambulatory electrocardiographic monitoring [4] that interest in this subject increased
[5].

My own interest in asymptomatic coronary artery disease began in the early 1970s and initially involved ECG responses during
exercise testing. Our first study was reported at the American
Heart Association meetings in 1975 [6] and was followed by a
review in 1977 [7] which described the unexpectedly vast scope
of the disorder. Introduction of the concept of a "defective
anginal warning system" soon followed with speculation as to its
causes and effect on prognosis [8]. It became apparent to me that
if this subject were to be investigated fully, a classification system
for asymptomatic coronary artery disease was necessary. Accordingly, in 1981 [9], we proposed that silent myocardial ischemia be
thought of as occurring in three types of patients with coronary
artery disease (Table 1). The first group consisted of persons who
were totally asymptomatic and the second group of persons who
were asymptomatic after an infarction. In addition, silent myocardial ischemia can be seen in patients with angina who also have
asymptomatic episodes. The key to this classification is in documentation of active ischemia; persons who have asymptomatic
coronary artery disease but are not experiencing active ischemia
are purposely not involved in this classification. Thus, someone
with an infarction, a totally occluded vessel and no ongoing
ischemia by objective criteria would be excluded.

The five major questions that were posed in the 1981 review [9] are still pertinent today and form the basis for this monograph, slightly modified. They are

1. What is the pathophysiologic basis of silent myocardial ischemia and silent myocardial infarction?

2. What is the prevalence of the different types of silent myocardial ischemia, and of silent myocardial infarction?

3. What are the most reliable noninvasive methods of detecting the syndrome of silent myocardial ischemia, and what are the indications for cardiac catheterization?

4. What is the prognosis of patients with silent myocardial ischemia and/or silent myocardial infarction?

5. How should silent myocardial ischemia be treated, if at all? Others have also posed similar questions [10].

The first attempt at answering these questions in a systematic way was in a seminar that appeared in 1983 in the *Journal of the American College of Cardiology* [11]. The present monograph represents a more comprehensive updating of that material as well as data from other sources, including a symposium on Silent Myocardial Ischemia held in Geneva, Switzerland, in 1984 under the auspices of the European Society of Cardiology [12]. Hopefully, by the time the reader finishes this most recent review of this syndrome, a clearer understanding of its pathophysiology, detection and management will emerge.

REFERENCES

1. M. D. Roseman. Painless myocardial infarction: A review of the literature and analysis of 220 cases. *Ann. Int. Med., 41*:1 (1954).

2. A. M. Master and A. M. Geller. The extent of completely asymptomatic coronary artery disease. *Am. J. Cardiol., 23*: 173 (1969).

3. V. F. Froelicher, F. G. Yanowitz, and A. J. Thompson. The correlation of coronary angiography and the electrocardiographic response to maximal treadmill testing in 76 asymptomatic men. *Circulation, 48*:597 (1973).

4. S. Stern and D. Tzivoni. Early detection of silent ischaemic heart disease by 24-hour electrocardiographic monitoring of active subjects. *Br. Heart J., 35*:481 (1974).

5. L. S. Gettes. Painless myocardial ischemia. *Chest*, *66*:612 (1974).
6. H. E. Lindsey and P. F. Cohn. "Silent" ischemia during and after exercise testing in patients with coronary artery disease (abstr). *Circulation*, *52*(Suppl 11):46 (1975).
7. P. F. Cohn. Severe asymptomatic coronary artery disease: A diagnostic, prognostic and therapeutic puzzle. *Am. J. Med.*, *62*:565 (1977).
8. P. F. Cohn. Silent myocardial ischemia in patients with a defective anginal warning system. *Am. J. Cardiol.*, *45*:697 (1980).
9. P. F. Cohn. Asymptomatic coronary artery disease: Pathophysiology, diagnosis, management. *Mod. Conc. Cardiovasc. Dis.*, *50*:55 (1981).
10. A. S. Iskandrian, B. L. Segal, and G. S. Anderson. Asymptomatic myocardial ischemia. *Arch. Int. Med.*, *141*:95 (1981).
11. P. F. Cohn. Introduction to Seminar on Asymptomatic Coronary Artery Disease. *J. Am. Coll. Cardiol.*, *3*:922 (1983).
12. W. Rutishauser and H. Roskamm, eds. *Silent Myocardial Ischemia*. Springer–Verlag, Berlin, 1984.

I
PATHOPHYSIOLOGY OF SILENT MYOCARDIAL ISCHEMIA

1
Cardiac Pain Mechanisms

Because pain is subjective, it cannot be readily investigated with the kinds of experimental models that are usually employed in laboratory settings. In those experimental pain studies that *can* be performed, some pain modalities are easier to assess than others. Somatic pain is one of the "easier" types, whereas visceral pain is harder to categorize experimentally. Therefore, cardiac pain, being

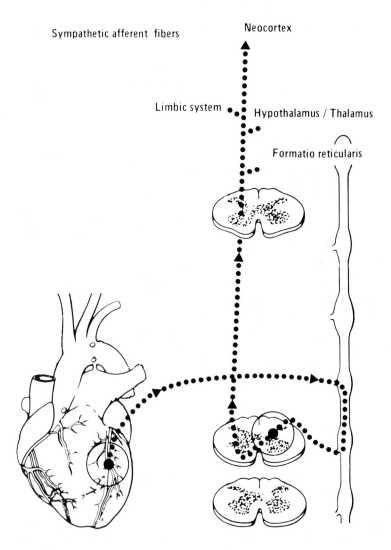

Figure 1   Mechanisms of cardiac pain. (From C. Droste and H. Roskamm, in *Silent Myocardial Ischemia* [W. Rutishauser and H. Roskamm, eds.] , Springer-Verlag, Berlin, 1984.)

visceral in nature, does not lend itself easily to reproducible studies in the animal laboratory.

I. NEUROANATOMY OF CARDIAC PAIN PATHWAYS

What has been established in the animal laboratory is the gross anatomy of cardiac nociceptive pathways [1]. The afferent fibers that run in the cardiac sympathetic nerves are usually thought of as the only essential pathway for the transmission of cardiac pain. The atria and ventricles are abundantly supplied with sympathetic sensory innervation; from the heart the sensory nerve endings connect to afferent fibers in cardiac nerve bundles which in turn connect to the upper five thoracic sympathetic ganglia and the upper five thoracic dorsal roots of the spinal cord (Figure 1). Within the spinal cord itself, impulses mediated by this sympathetic afferent route probably converge with impulses from somatic thoracic structures onto the same ascending spinal neurons. This would be the basis for cardiac referred pain, i.e., pain referred to the chest wall, arm, back, etc. In addition to this "convergence–projection theory" (first proposed by Ruch [2] over 30 years ago and more recently supported by Foreman's studies [3]), the contribution of vagal afferent fibers must be acknowledged or else we have no explanation for cardiac pain referred to the jaw and neck. How these vagal fibers are activated remains unclear.

II. THEORIES OF CARDIAC PAIN

The links between disease of the coronary arteries and cardiac pain go back to the time of Heberden's original descriptions of the clinical picture of angina pectoris. Early writers believed that coronary spasm was common and that interruption in blood supply could produce pain. Lewis [4] has noted that Potain was the first to draw the analogy between pain arising from ischemic myocardium and an ischemic limb. But what was the actual "trigger" that stimulated the sensory nerve endings? Lewis proposed that a chemical pain stimulus was involved, the so-called "factor P" produced by exercise-induced ischemia. Others proposed that anoxia itself was the cause of the pain. The "trigger" is still unclear. At one time, a mechanical stimulus (stretching of the coronary arteries) was also proposed as the cause of the pain even when ischemia

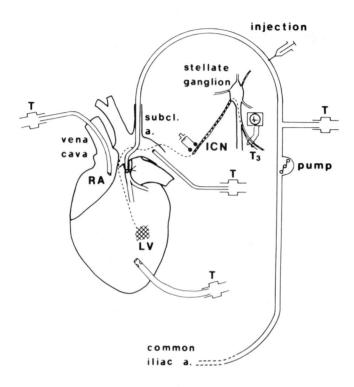

Figure 2   Schema of the experimental model used in the cat for recording impulse activity of single afferent ventricular sympathetic nonmyelinated nerve fibers. The conduction velocity of the recorded fiber is determined by stimulating the inferior cardiac nerve (ICN) or the surrounding tissues. The extracorporeal perfusion circuit allows the interruption of the left main coronary artery flow or the intracoronary administration of chemical substances without direct manipulation of the heart. RA = right atrium; LV = left ventricle; T = transducer. (From A. Malliani, *Rev. Physiol. Biochem. Pharmacol.*, *94*:11, 1982.)

itself was not induced. This was suggested after watching the behavior of laboratory animals whose coronary arteries were stretched.

More recently, the nociceptive (pain-bearing) function of the cardiac sympathetic fibers has itself been challenged, especially by Malliani [5–7]. Malliani notes that the two main hypotheses for the peripheral (somatic) manifestation of pain are the "intensity"

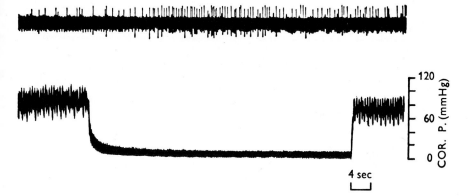

Figure 3   Effect of myocardial ischemia on an afferent unit in the inferior cardiac nerve. The sudden fall in coronary pressure (Cor. P. in mmHg) occurred when the inflow was stopped. There was some background activity which showed a marked increase during ischemia. (From A. M. Brown and A. Malliani, *J. Physiol.*, *212*: 685, 1971.)

and "specificity" hypotheses. The "intensity" hypothesis assumes that pain results from an excessive stimulation of receptive structures. The "specificity" hypothesis postulates that pain is conceived as a specific sensation by excitation of a well-defined nociceptive system that responds to noxious stimuli. Malliani poses the question: Do specific cardiac nociceptors exist? Are there hundreds of cardiac nerve fibers exclusively designed for signaling higher centers about certain kinds of coronary emergencies?

III. EXPERIMENTAL STUDIES

Electrophysiologic studies of the afferent fibers that are most likely to convey cardiac nociception (the ventricular fibers) evaluated these fibers for absence of spontaneous impulse activity, unresponsiveness to normal physiologic hemodynamic stimuli, and the ability to respond to stimuli of pathophysiologic significance. In Malliani's experiments, multifiber recordings were obtained from afferent sympathetic fibers (Figure 2). As indicated in Figure 3, excitation could be demonstrated during interruption of coronary

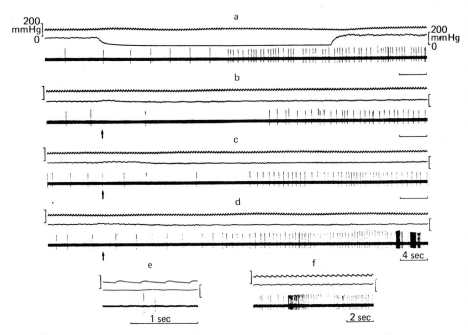

Figure 4   Activity of an afferent sympathetic unmyelinated nerve
fiber with a left ventricular ending. Tracings represent from top to
bottom: systemic arterial pressure, coronary perfusion pressure,
nerve impulse activity (cathode-ray oscilloscope recordings). a.
Interruption of the left main coronary artery perfusion; b. intracoronary administration, beginning at the arrow, of bradykinin
5 ng/kg; c. intracoronary administration of bradykinin 10 ng/kg;
d. intracoronary administration of bradykinin 30 ng/kg; e. electrical stimulation of the left inferior cardiac nerve activating the afferent fiber to calculate the conduction velocity; f. mechanical prob-
ing, marked by a bar, of an area of the external surface of the left
ventricle. (From F. Lombardi, P. Della Bella, R. Casati, and A.
Malliani. *Circ. Res.*, *48*:69, 1981. Reproduced with the permission of the American Heart Association.)

blood flow. In the early experiments, recruitment of a few silent
units, i.e., with obvious background discharge, could be demonstrated by computer assisted techniques. This recruitment suggested to Malliani and co-workers that specific cardiac nociceptors
were present. Reexamination of the data in later experiments [6]

cast doubts about this interpretation in light of the animal preparation used. In the preparation, the spinal cord was transsected and the baseline arterial pressure was low enough to "artificially" reduce the normal background discharge of the fibers. In his most recent experiments [8] using coronary occlusion or the intracoronary administration of bradykinin — a naturally occurring substance that is believed to play a role in the genesis of cardiac pain — no recruitment of silent afferent units could be demonstrated (Figure 4). Thus, whether myelinated or not, the ventricular afferent fibers always possessed some degree of spontaneous impulse activity and a responsiveness to normal hemodynamic stimuli. Malliani concluded that the sensitivity to both mechanical and chemical stimuli, such as bradykinin, was not unique, as others [9] claimed.

Malliani has also commented on behavior of conscious animals exposed to intense excitation of cardiovascular sympathetic fibers. In one of his experiments, the thoracic aorta was stretched via an implanted and inflatable rubber cylinder [10]. A mechanical stimulus elicited a pressor reflex without any pain. In the other experiment, bradykinin was injected directly into a branch of the left coronary artery that had previously been cannulated. Despite pressor responses, there was no pain (Figure 5). However, when the same experiment was performed three days after surgery, the animal was obviously in pain; the surgery had "facilitated" the cardiac pain. Under chronic conditions with an implanted occluder, Theroux et al. [11] reported pain responses are variable. Thus, Malliani has concluded that no specific cardiac nociceptive apparatus could be confirmed. Rather, the "intensity" hypothesis appears a more valid explanation.

IV. RELATION OF EXPERIMENTAL STUDIES TO THE CLINICAL SETTING

How does the "intensity" pain mechanism relate to the clinical setting and particularly to the occurrence of silent myocardial ischemia? Sufficient levels of afferent impulses must be reached and an appropriate activation of the central ascending pathways must be established before a breakthrough can occur and there is a conscious perception of pain. The level of impulses may be influenced by hypertension and tachycardia preceding the ischemia episodes — the more general the cardiac sympathetic afferent dis-

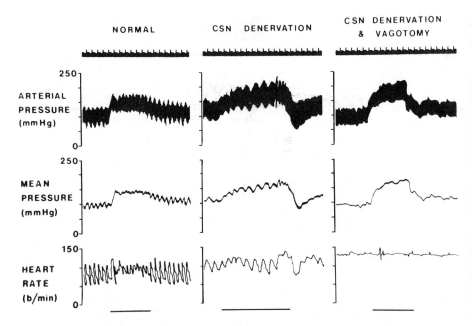

Figure 5   Reflex effects of aortic distension (indicated by the bottom bars) on systemic arterial pressure and heart rate in a conscious dog. The left panel depicts the control response, the middle panel the response after carotid sinoaortic denervation and the right panel the response after further sectioning of both vagi. Note the progressive increase of the pressor response that follows the denervation procedures. "Pain" (i.e., agitation, etc.) was not observed in any of these experiments. (From M. Pagani, P. Pizzinelli, M. Bergamaschi, and A. Malliani. *Circ. Res.*, *50*:125, 1982.)

charge, the more likely the intensity of discharges will reach the critical threshold necessary to convert a receptive process (nociception) into a conscious experience (angina pectoris). By not reaching this critical threshold, ischemia remains "silent." Whether this is the only mechanism is unresolved, but at the present time it seems a reasonable hypothesis.

V. CONCLUSIONS

The gross anatomy of the cardiac pain pathway appears to be well worked out, but whether the cardiac sympathetic fibers function as true nociceptors has been seriously questioned. Despite decades of speculation, the actual chemical "trigger" is also still unclear.

REFERENCES

1. J. C. White. Cardiac pain. Anatomic pathways and physiologic mechanisms. *Circulation, 16*:644 (1957).
2. T. C. Ruch. Pathophysiology of pain. In *A Textbook of Physiology* (J. F. Fulton, ed.), W. B. Saunders Co., Philadelphia, 1955, p. 358.
3. R. D. Foreman, C. A. Ohata, and K. D. Gerhart. Neural mechanisms underlying cardiac pain. In *Neural Mechanisms in Cardiac Arrhythmias* (P. J. Schwartz, A. M. Brown, A. Malliani, and A. Zanchetti, eds.), Raven Press, New York, 1978, p. 191.
4. T. Lewis. Pain in muscular ischemia — Its relation to anginal pain. *Arch. Intern Med., 49*:713 (1932).
5. A. Malliani and F. Lombardia. Consideration of the fundamental mechanisms eliciting cardiac pain. *Am. Heart J., 103*:575 (1982).
6. A. Malliani. Cardiovascular sympathetic afferent fibers. *Rev. Physiol. Biochem. Pharmacol., 94*:11 (1982).
7. A. M. Brown and A. Malliani. Spinal sympathetic reflexes initiated by coronary receptors. *J. Physiol., 212*:685 (1971).
8. F. Lombardi, P. Della Bella, R. Casati, and A. Malliani. Effects of intracoronary administration of bradykinin on the impulse activity of afferent sympathetic unmyelinated fibers with left ventricular endings in the cat. *Circ. Res., 48*:69 (1981).
9. D. G. Baker, H. M. Coleridge, J. C. G. Coleridge, and T. Terndrum. Search for a cardiac nociceptor: Stimulation by bradykinin of sympathetic afferent nerve endings in the heart of the cat. *J. Physiol., 306*:519 (1980).
10. M. Pagani, P. Pizzinelli, M. Bergamaschi, and A. Malliani. A positive feedback sympathetic pressor reflex during stretch of the thoracic aorta in conscious dogs. *Circ. Res., 50*:125 (1982).
11. P. Theroux, J. Ross, D. Franklin, W. S. Kemper, and S. Sassayama. Regional myocardial function in the conscious dog during acute coronary occlusion and responses to morphine, propranolol, nitroglycerin, and lidocaine. *Circulation, 53*:302 (1976).

2
Alterations in Sensibility to Pain in Patients with Silent Myocardial Ischemia

Why pain is not present during episodes of silent myocardial ischemia is unclear; one possible mechanism is an alteration in the patient's sensibility to pain, either centrally or peripherally.

Table 1   Comparison of Selected Medical Variables Measured in
Patients with Symptomatic and Asymptomatic Myocardial Ischemia

	Myocardial Ischemia	
	Symptomatic (n = 22)	Asymptomatic (n = 20)
1 vessel disease	9 ⎫	3 ⎫
2 vessel disease	3 ⎬ 2.1 ± 0.9	3 ⎬ 2.5 ± 0.8
3 vessel disease	10 ⎭	14 ⎭
Friesinger score	8.6 ± 3.1	10.4 ± 2.6
Ejection fraction (%)	60 ± 16	58 ± 12
Heart volume (ml)	816 ± 142	856 ± 220
Heart volume related to body weight (ml/kg)	10.9 ± 1.2	11.1 ± 2.5
Previous myocardial infarction (no. of patients)	17	16
Risk factors		
Age (yr)	51 ± 5.8	52 ± 9.6
Smoking	17	10
Hypertension (> 140 > 95 mm Hg)	8	8
Diabetes	1	2
Cholesterol (mg/dl)	240 ± 40	237 ± 65
Triglycerides (mg/dl)	195 ± 83	174 ± 79

All data are = standard deviation values.
Differences between the symptomatic and asymptomatic groups for each variable were not significant.
(From C. Droste and H. Roskamm. Experimental pain measurement in patients with asymptomatic myocardial ischemia. *J. Am. Coll. Cardiol.*, *1*:940, 1983.)

I. STUDIES OF PAIN THRESHOLD AND PAIN PERCEPTION

The most thorough investigation of this subject to date is that of Droste and Roskamm [1]. These investigators studied 42 men (mean age 51 years). All patients had angiographically confirmed coronary artery disease, i.e., ≥ 75% stenosis in at least one major coronary artery. In addition, they all had > 1.0 mm ST segment depression on multiple exercise studies. Patients were divided into two groups depending on the occurrence of angina pectoris during the exercise tests. Factors such as digitalis medication, hykolemia, valvular heart disease, etc. that could have been responsible for specious ST segment depression were excluded. All patients had normal neurologic examinations. There were 20 patients in the asymptomatic group; 16 had ECG evidence of prior infarction, but only 6 had pain with the infarction. Furthermore, 16 of the patients had no angina during everyday activity; the other 5 had complained of pain in the past. By contrast, in the symptomatic group (22 patients), only 2 of 17 patients who had prior infarctions had no pain with the infarctions. Distribution of coronary risk factors was similar in both groups, as were angiographic features (Table 1).

Droste and Roskamm studied three different modalities of pain perception. The first was an electrical pain threshold test in which the magnitude of pain current applied to the thigh was evaluated [2]. The value of threshold was reported according to the degree of electrical current used (in mA). The second test was a standard cold pressor test in which patient's left arm was submerged in water cooled at $4°C$. The third test was a modified form of the submaximal effort tourniquet technique in which the working muscle of the left arm is stressed [3]. The end point in the first test was the actual amount of electrical current needed to produce pain. In the other two tests, the time that elapsed before the patient perceived pain, or was no longer able to tolerate pain, was measured. The results of these studies showed striking differences when the two groups were compared. For example, when pain threshold was determined, symptomatic patients demonstrated a mean electrical pain threshold of 0.57 mA (Figure 1, top). This finding is in agreement with other studies performed in healthy men in which 0.55 mA was the average value. Asymptomatic patients had a much wider range of values with a mean value of 1.04 mA. During the cold pressor tests, asymptomatic patients showed much greater values for pain tolerance than did symptomatic patients (Figure 2, bottom). Pain thresholds showed a similar trend, but the differences were not statistically significant. During the arm muscle ischemic pain test, asymptomatic patients had a higher pain threshold and pain tolerance than symptomatic patients, though only the latter difference achieved statistical significance (Figure 3). In addition, asymptomatic patients rated a high stimulus as actually being less intense than did the symptomatic patients. (This was also true in the cold pressor test.)

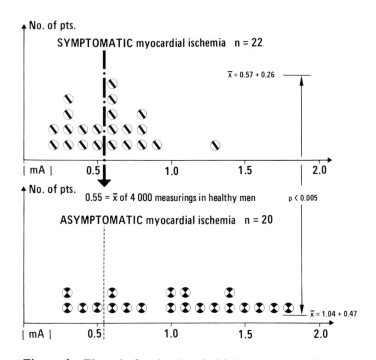

Figure 1   Electrical pain threshold in symptomatic and asymptomatic patients. (From C. Droste and H. Roskamm. *J. Am. Coll. Cardiol.*, *1*:940, 1983.)

II. CLINICAL FEATURES THAT MAY EXPLAIN ABSENCE OF PAIN

Droste and Roskamm discussed the results of their study at some length. They evaluated three arguments put forth as possible explanations for the lack of pain. The first has to do with destruction of nociceptive pathways by infarction, diffuse ischemia or some type of neuropathy. In these patients, however, the frequency of myocardial infarctions, extensive multivessel disease, diabetes or alcoholism was similar in both the symptomatic and asymptomatic subgroups. The authors pointed out that only radical surgical procedures — transplantation, autotransplantation, plexectomy — could sufficiently denervate a heart so that angina became absent. The authors also felt that their study amply demonstrated that

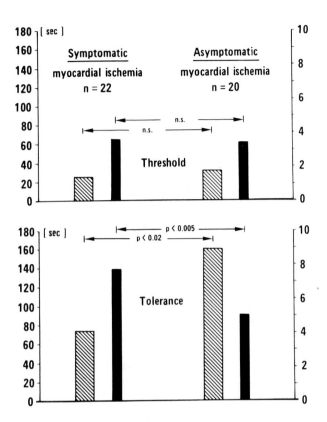

Figure 2   Cold pressor test: group differences for threshold and
tolerance levels. (Hatched columns = stimulus intensity; solid
columns = subjective experience of pain.) (From C. Droste and
H. Roskamm. *J. Am. Coll. Cardiol.*, *1*:940, 1983.)

the intensity of ischemia is not necessarily reduced in asymptomatic patients. They based this on the finding that the degree of
ischemia — as determined by ST depression — was comparable in
both groups. (We will comment further on this factor — the
amount of myocardium at jeopardy — in a subsequent chapter.)
Thus, they concluded that the hyposensibility to pain in general
that they reported best differentiated the asymptomatic from
the symptomatic patients. This supported earlier, less quantita-

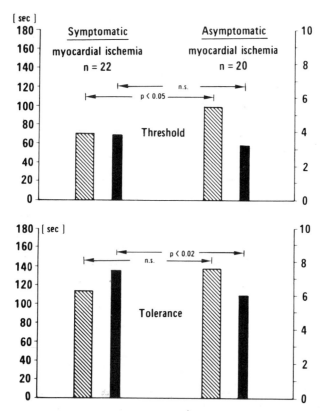

Figure 3   Ischemic pain test in the arm. (Hatched columns =
stimulus intensity; solid columns = subjective experience of pain.)
(From C. Droste and H. Roskamm. *J. Am. Coll. Cardiol.*, *1*:940,
1983.)

tive data from studies of patients with silent myocardial infarction
[4].*

The authors then posed the question as to which mechanisms
were involved in the decreased sensibility to pain: pain-discrimi-
nating ability versus individual response tendencies that categorize
a stimulus as pain. The authors felt that some of their data,

---

*Pain mechanisms in silent myocardial infarctions will be discussed further in
Chapter 7.

especially that dealing with the differences in electrically determined pain thresholds and thresholds for ischemic pain, supported the former mechanism. But the tendency for asymptomatic patients to rate painful stimuli as less intense — and thus tolerate the stimulus much longer — argues also for a difference in response tendencies. The two factors are not necessarily independent of each other.

III. POSSIBLE ROLE OF ENDORPHINS

Could endorphic mechanisms influence the difference in pain responses? Normally, varying concentrations of these opioidlike substances exist in plasma and cerebrospinal fluid and may be important in mediating pain sensitivity [5]. VanRijn and Dobkin [6] reported that injection of the opioid-antagonist naloxone precipitated angina earlier during exercise-induced ischemia than a placebo. However, they only tested 5 patients. We have been unable to reproduce these results in 8 symptomatic patients, nor have we been able to use this agent to precipitate angina during treadmill exercise tests in 9 patients with documented silent myocardial ischemia [7]. Patients were given 2 mg of naloxone intravenously prior to exercise tests and results compared to placebo tests. Duration of exercise tests in asymptomatic patients (to 1 mm of ST depression) were as follows: control 412 ± 43 sec, placebo 382 ± 113 sec, naloxone 360 ± 110 sec (pNS). In a similar study, Ellestad and Kuan [8] reported on their findings in 10 men with asymptomatic but positive stress tests. These men were given naloxone, 2 mg intravenously, and the tests repeated. No chest pain was reported by any patient and naloxone did not significantly alter exercise duration, heart rate, blood pressure or ST segment changes compared to the control test (Table 2).

Droste and Roskamm have reported results different from those cited above. They studied 60 patients [9] in a manner similar to their earlier studies in 42 patients [1]. The 60 patients were evenly divided between those with and those without asymptomatic ischemia. The asymptomatic patients had reproducible asymptomatic manifestations of myocardial ischemia in several exercise tests. Mean ST depression was 3.8 mm (0.38 mV). Factors that could have indicated false-positive ST segment depression such as other forms of heart disease or cardiac medications were excluded.

Table 2 Results of Treadmill Stress Testing in 10 Men

Pt	Age (yr)	History of MI	Medications	Maximal Treadmill Exercise							
				Duration (sec)		Heart Rate (beats/min)		Blood Pressure (mm Hg)		Maximal ST Depression (mm)	
				C	N	C	N	C	N	C	N
1	63	+	0	705	720	160	160	168/50	180/70	6	7
2	53	0	Propranolol	600	600	150	159	138/78	150/90	3	2
3	57	0	0	420	420	152	170	180/70	160/70	5	5
4	60	+	Nifedipine	290	300	128	127	180/80	175/80	3	4
5	67	0	Propranolol	240	300	140	140	160/70	160/70	4	4
6	66	0	Propranolol	600	600	142	123	180/90	140/70	6	5
7	65	+	Nifedipine	560	540	160	164	176/90	180/90	5	5
8	61	0	0	480	420	165	150	150/80	160/70	4	4
9	75	0	Propranolol	420	420	131	110	180/90	190/80	5	5
10	53	0	Diltiazem	420	480	146	147	160/80	150/68	2	2
Mean	62			473.5	480	147	145	167/79	164/76	4.3	4.3
± SD	± 6.8			± 145	± 136	± 12	± 19	± 15/± 12	± 16/± 9	± 1.3	± 1.5

C = control; MI = myocardial infarction; N = naloxone infusion; SD = standard deviation; + = present; 0 = absent.
(From M. H. Ellestad and P. Kuan. Am. J. Cardiol., 54:982, 1984.)

Table 3 Parameters of Exercise Testing Before and After
Naloxone Injection in 10 Patients with Asymptomatic Myocardial
Ischemia

			Before Injection (Placebo)	After Injection
Rest	Heart rate		72	70
	Blood pressure	systolic	129	127
		diastolic	83	83
Maximal effort	Watts		100	100
	Heart rate		129	128
	Blood pressure	systolic	176	175
		diastolic	103	102
	ST (mV)		0.34	0.32

(From C. Droste and H. Roskamm. Pain measurement and pain modification
by naloxone in patients with asymptomatic myocardial ischemia. In *Silent
Myocardial Ischemia* [W. Rutishauser and H. Roskamm, eds.], Springer–Verlag,
Berlin, 1984.)

Most of these patients did not have angina during everyday activities and most had had prior myocardial infarctions. All patients
had angiographically proven coronary artery disease. A control
group of 30 patients with symptomatic coronary artery disease
had less ST segment depression during exercise testing (2.2 mm),
but other selected mechanical variables showed no difference between the two groups. These variables included age, smoking history and other clinical features, as well as angiographic measurements such as number of vessels diseased, ejection fraction, etc.
The three different pain-receptive modalities employed in their
previous study [1] were repeated in this study with similar results.
In 10 asymptomatic patients, the tests were repeated following
intravenous injection of 2 mg of saline and again after a placebo
injection. As indicated in Table 3, there were no differences in
parameters of exercise testing (maximum effort, heart rate, blood
pressure or ST segment depression) between the placebo tests and
those employing naloxone. Two of the ten patients developed

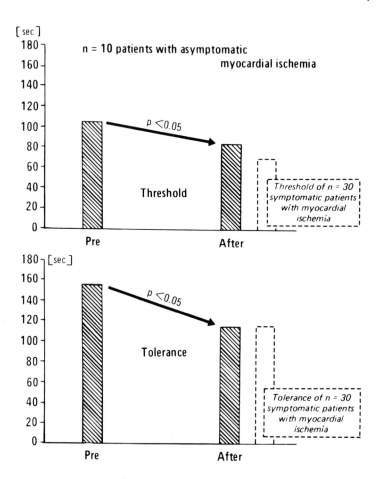

Figure 4   Ischemic pain test in the arm. Values before and after naloxone injection in 10 patients with asymptomatic myocardial ischemia. (From C. Droste and H. Roskamm. Pain measurement and pain modification by naloxone in patients with asymptomatic myocardial ischemia. In *Silent Myocardial Ischemia* [W. Rutishauser and H. Roskamm, eds.], Springer–Verlag, Berlin, 1984.)

angina during the naloxone test, though one required 4 mg of the drug before this response was elicited. The most striking finding was during the ischemic pain test in which arm ischemia is produced by a tourniquet. Both the threshold to pain and tolerance to it were significantly altered after naloxone administration (Figure 4). The investigators concluded that the result lent support to their previous work showing a differential sensitivity to pain and suggested a possible role for endorphic mechanisms in silent myocardial ischemia. Others have reported that endorphin secretion may be the mechanism whereby transcutaneous electrical nerve stimulation reduces angina [10]. Thus, cardiac pain may indeed be influenced by endorphins, as Droste and Roskamm concluded. There is no mention in their work as to whether they could confirm Van Rijn and Rabkin's exercise studies in symptomatic patients.

In summary, the evidence linking endorphins to silent myocardial ischemia is inconclusive. It is possible that there are naloxone-insensitive opioid receptors, or that opioid peptides other than endorphins are responsible for inhibition of angina in these patients. It is also possible that a 2-mg dose of naloxone was inadequate to antagonize high levels of endorphins. However, most studies of general pain responses have demonstrated physiologic and pharmacologic effects in the 0.4- to 2.0-mg dose range.

IV. CONCLUSIONS

There is evidence to suggest that some patients with silent myocardial ischemia have an altered sensibility to certain types of pain. Whether endorphins can influence this hyposensibility is unproven.

REFERENCES

1. C. Droste and H. Roskamm. Experimental pain measurement in patients with asymptomatic myocardial ischemia. *J. Am. Coll. Cardiol.*, 1:940 (1983).
2. S. L. H. Notermans. Measurement of the pain threshold determined by electrical stimulation and its clinical application. In *Pain, Clinical and Experimental Perspectives* (M. Weisenberg, ed.), Mosby, St. Louis, pp. 72–87 (1975).

3. P. A. Moore, G. H. Duncan, D. S. Scott, J. M. Gress, and J. N. Ghia. The submaximum effort tourniquet test: its use in evaluating experimental and chronic pain. *Pain*, *6*:382 (1979).
4. P. Procacei, M. Zoppi, L. Padeletii, and M. Maresca. Myocardial infarction without pain. A study of the sensory function of the upper limbs. *Pain*, *2*:309 (1976).
5. M. S. Buchsbaum, G. C. Davies, R. Coppola, and D. Naber. Opiate pharmacology and individual differences. I. Phychophysical pain measurements. *Pain*, *10*:367 (1981).
6. T. VanRijn and S. W. Rabkin. Effect of naloxone, a specific opioid antagonist, on exercise induced angina pectoris (Abstr). *Circulation*, *64*(Suppl 4):149 (1981).
7. P. F. Cohn, R. Patcha, S. Singh, S. C. Vlay, G. Mallis, and W. Lawson. Effect of naloxone on exercise tests in patients with symptomatic and silent myocardial ischemia (abstr). *Clin. Res.*, *33*:177A (1985).
8. M. H. Ellestad and P. Kuan. Naloxone and asymptomatic ischemia. Failure to induce angina during exercise testing. *Am. J. Cardiol. 54*:928 (1984).
9. C. Droste and H. Roskamm. Pain measurement and pain modification by naloxone in patients with asymptomatic myocardial ischemia. In *Silent Myocardial Ischemia* (W. Rutishauser and H. Roskamm, eds.), Springer–Verlag, Berlin, 1984, pp. 14–23.
10. C. Mannheimer, C–A. Carlsson, H. Emanuelsson, A. Vedin, A. F. Waagstein, and C. Wilhelmsson. The effects of transcutaneous electrical nerve stimulation in patients with severe angina pectoris. *Circulation*, *71*:308 (1985).

3
The Sequence of Events During Episodes of Myocardial Ischemia
Where does pain fit in?

In order to appreciate the pathophysiologic significance of silent myocardial ischemia, an understanding of the sequence of events leading up to the occurrence of pain during episodes of myocardial ischemia is important. The use of intracardiac catheterization

techniques has greatly facilitated these kinds of studies and several
reports published in the past five years are worth commenting on
in detail.

I. ATRIAL PACING STUDIES

Markham et al. [1] used atrial pacing to assess symptomatic electrocardiographic, metabolic and hemodynamic alterations in 28
patients, 18 with coronary artery disease and 10 with normal coronary arteriograms. Before pacing, arterial and coronary sinus
blood samples were obtained for quantitation of lactate and oxygen content. Left ventricular systolic and end-diastolic pressures
and left ventricular dP/dt (a contractility index) were recorded,
and a radionuclide ventriculogram obtained. The measurements
were repeated at the termination of the peak atrial pacing rate.
Previous studies had indicated that pacing-induced chest pain was
a reliable marker for underlying coronary artery disease. This was
not found in the study of Markham and colleagues. Similarly,
postpacing electrocardiograms offered only modest sensitivity and
specificity in the identification of pacing-induced ischemia. Lactate production in this study — as in others — was a specific indication of ischemia. Lactate production reflects anerobic glycolysis
in the ischemic tissue with resultant release of lactate into the
coronary sinus effluent. However, lactate production was not a
sensitive indicator of left ventricular dysfunction. What of the
pacing-induced increase in left ventricular filling pressure? This
also had been found in prior studies to be a common occurrence
during angina. In the present study, a more than 5 mmHg rise in
left ventricular end-diastolic pressure was found to be a specific
but not very sensitive indicator of pacing induced left ventricular
dysfunction. The latter was defined as a decrease of 5% or more
in left ventricular ejection fraction combined with new segmental
wall abnormalities. This alteration in left ventricular ejection fraction is commonly attributed to ischemia and, therefore, was used
as the "gold standard" for myocardial ischemia in the Markham
study.

II. EXERCISE STUDIES

To more specifically address the issue of *sequence* of these events,
Upton and colleagues [2] used radionuclide ventriculography in

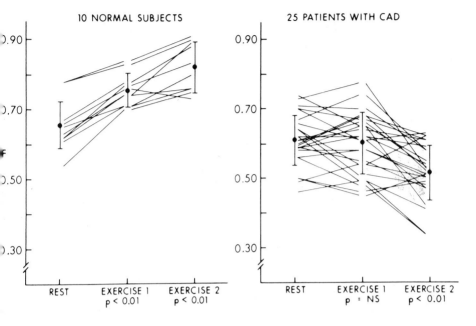

Figure 1   Changes in ejection fraction (EF) from rest to the first
level of exercise (exercise 1) and the second level (exercise 2) in 10
normal subjects and the 25 patients with coronary artery disease
(CAD). (From M. T. Upton, S. K. Rerych, G. E. Newman, S. Port,
F. R. Cobb, and R. H. Jones. *Circulation*, *62*:341, 1980.)

25 coronary artery disease patients and 10 normal controls to
evaluate left ventricular dysfunction. These investigators pro-
voked ischemia with two levels of an upright bicycle exercise test.
The first radionuclide study during exercise was performed before
the onset of ST segment depression and the second one after its
appearance. As indicated in Figure 1, the mean ejection fraction
increased in the normal subjects during the first level of exercise
but remained unchanged (an abnormal response) in the patients
with coronary artery disease. At the second level of exercise, the
control group continued to show an increase, while in the coronary artery disease group there was now a frank decrease for the
group as a whole and all patients showed an abnormal response.
Wall motion patterns showed a similar trend (Figure 2). A regional

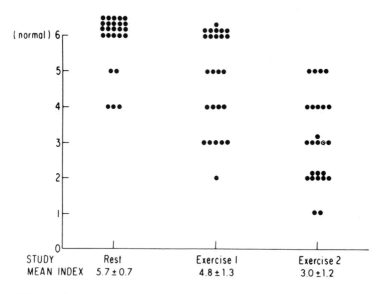

Figure 2   Regional wall motion index in 25 patients with coronary artery disease at rest, exercise 1 and exercise 2. (From M. T. Upton, S. K. Rerych, G. E. Newman, S. Port, F. R. Cobb, and R. H. Jones. *Circulation*, *62*:341, 1980. Reproduced with permission of the American Heart Association.)

wall motion index was used to assess these changes. At the first level of exercise, 14 of the coronary patients (56%) developed a new wall motion abnormality or demonstrated progression in a preexisting defect at rest. At the second level of exercise, wall motion was abnormal in all patients. Nine of the twenty-five patients with coronary artery disease did not experience angina during these studies. Thus, this study concluded that angina pectoris and ST segment shifts on the electrocardiogram are frequently *late* manifestations of myocardial ischemia.

III. CONTINUOUS HEMODYNAMIC MONITORING

Possibly the single most important of these studies emanated from Maseri's laboratory. This study by Chierchia et al. [3] is important because of the intensive invasive and noninvasive monitoring

Table 1   ST-T Changes During 137 Ischemic Episodes

Pt No.	ST↑		ST↓		T↑	
	P	A	P	A	P	A
1	1	16				55
2	2	1				
3			1	1		
4	1	4				31
5	3				2	18
6	1			1		
	7	21	1	2	2	104

Abbreviations: P = painful episodes; A = asymptomatic episodes; ST↑ = ST segment elevation; ST↓ = ST segment depression; T↑ = pseudonormalization of T waves.
(From S. Chierchia, C. Brunelli, I. Simonetti, M. Lazzari, and A. Maseri. *Circulation*, *61*:759, 1980.)

that the six patients in the study underwent. These six patients were admitted to the coronary care unit because of transient, recurrent episodes of angina at rest with typical ST-T changes. To document the location and direction of ST segment changes, 12-lead ECG tracings were recorded in each patient during the course of several angina attacks. In addition to electrocardiographic monitoring, the left ventricular or aortic pressure was continuously monitored, as well as the coronary sinus oxygen saturation. The latter was assumed to reflect changes in myocardial blood flow, provided the arterial oxygen content and the myocardial oxygen consumption remained constant. Thirty-one episodes of ST segment or T wave abnormalities (most involving ST segment elevation in these mainly Prinzmetal angina patients) were recorded (Table 1). Only eight episodes were accompanied by typical angina pain. Although the ischemic episodes were accompanied by different hemodynamic patterns in individual patients, some common features were striking. Pain when present occurred 50–120 seconds *after* the onset of ST-T wave changes. The authors concluded that pain did not appear to be a reliable and sensitive marker of transient, acute myocardial ischemia. In none of these

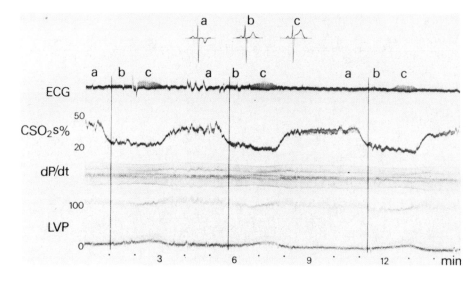

Figure 3   Low-speed playback (paper speed 0.3 mm/sec) of ECG, coronary sinus O_2 saturation (CSO_2S), left ventricular pressure (LVP) and dP/dt during three successive asymptomatic episodes recorded over a period of about 15 minutes. At the top are electrocardiographic patterns (lead V_2) in resting conditions (a), at the onset (b) and at the peak (c) of the ischemic episode. Vertical lines correspond to the onset of the ST–T changes. A sharp drop of CSO_2S (denoting reduction in coronary blood flow) consistently precedes the onset of ECG and hemodynamic changes. (From S. Chierchia, I. Simonetti, M. Lazzari, and A. Maseri. *Circulation*, *61*:759, 1980. Reproduced with permission of the American Heart Association.)

patients with rest angina were the ST–T changes preceded by consistent increases in the hemodynamic determinants of myocardial oxygen consumption (such as increased heart rate or blood pressure). Hemodynamic changes reflecting acute left ventricular functional impairment did occur before ST changes but even earlier changes usually occurred in the coronary sinus oxygen saturation. This presumably reflected decreased myocardial blood flow. Figures 3 and 4 depict the sequence of events: primary reduction in coronary blood flow, fall in left ventricular systolic pressure and left ventricular dP/dt, the same contractility index

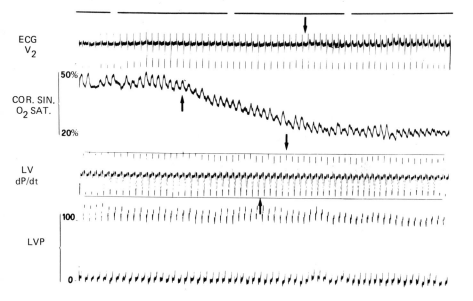

Figure 4 High-speed playback (paper speed 10 mm/sec) of the transient phase of an ischemic episode characterized by peaking of T waves. Arrows indicate the onset of change for each recorded parameter. A drop in CSO_2S (denoting reduction in coronary blood flow) precedes the onset of ECG and hemodynamic changes. (From S. Chierchia, C. Brunelli, I. Simonetti, M. Lazzari, and A. Maseri. *Circulation, 61*:759, 1980. Reproduced with permission of the American Heart Association.)

used by Markham et al. [1], and a rise in left ventricular enddiastolic pressure, and then ST–T changes. Pain was the final event, when it occurred. The truly ischemic nature of these episodes was confirmed by thallium-201 scintigrams during painless episodes in four patients that showed perfusion defects relative to control tracings.

IV. TRANSIENT CORONARY ARTERY OBSTRUCTION DURING BALLOON ANGIOPLASTY

Recently, Sigwart and colleagues [4] have shed additional light on the sequence of ischemic events by carefully monitoring several

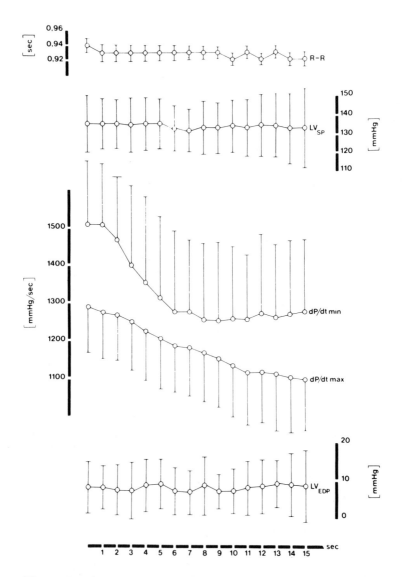

Figure 5   Heart rate (R–R), left ventricular systolic pressure (LV$_{sp}$)
dP/dt min, dP/dt max, and left ventricular end-diastolic pressure
(LV$_{EDP}$) during the first 15-sec coronary balloon obstruction in 12
patients (mean ± 1 SD). (From U. Sigwart, M. Grbic, M. Payot, J.-J.
Goy, A. Essinger, and A. Fischer. In *Silent Myocardial Ischemia* [W.
Rutishauser and H. Roskamm, eds.], Springer-Verlag, Berlin, 1984.)

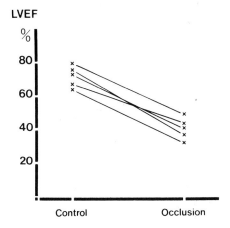

LVEF

Figure 6   Left ventricular ejection fraction (LVEF) measured with biplane cineangiography before and during coronary balloon occlusion. (From U. Sigwart, M. Grbic, M. Payot, J.-J. Goy, A. Essinger, and A. Fischer. In *Silent Myocardial Ischemia* [W. Rutishauser and H. Roskamm, eds.], Springer–Verlag, Berlin, 1984.)

variables during balloon obstruction of the coronary arteries in humans. This technique — the key part of the transluminal coronary angioplasty procedure — allows the onset of ischemia to be precisely defined in a controlled setting. In 12 patients, one catheter was placed in the pulmonary artery, and a high-fidelity micromanometer was placed in the left ventricle via the transseptal approach. The time of coronary occlusion was identified by a sudden pressure drop at the distal end of the balloon catheter. Duration of the balloon occlusion was adjusted according to the alteration in the contractility and relaxation variables that were measured. Left ventricular dimensional changes were obtained in 5 patients with M-mode echocardiography and in 5 patients with biplane angiography. The time course of various hemodynamic changes is shown in Figure 5. Heart rate and blood pressure changes were small during the first 15 seconds of the balloon occlusion (which usually involved the left anterior descending coronary artery), but dP/dt max and dP/dt min (the latter an index of relaxation) fell. Left ventricular end-diastolic pressure changed little. Ejection fraction measured 10 seconds after occlusion in five patients was reduced by over one-third of the control value (Figure 6). Angina, when it occurred, was later than 25

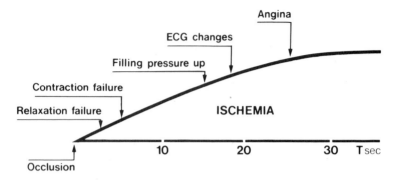

Figure 7   Appearance of events during transient coronary occlusion. (From U. Sigwart, M. Grbic, M. Payot, J.-J. Goy, A. Essinger, and A. Fischer. In *Silent Myocardial Ischemia* [W. Rutishauser and H. Roskamm, eds.], Springer–Verlag, Berlin, 1984.)

seconds after balloon occlusion and was usually preceeded by ECG changes. Figure 7 shows the sequence of events over the course of the first 30 seconds after occlusion. It was of interest that the relaxation parameters were the most sensitive of all the variables. This confirmed earlier reports in experimental animals, as well as other studies of transluminal angioplasty in man. The authors concluded that "ischemia in conscious man is always characterized by a transition period during which it remains silent." During the silent stage of the ischemic event, the signs of left ventricular dysfunction may be drastic, as others have also shown [5]. As we shall see from other clinical studies in subsequent chapters, the transition to a symptomatic stage does not necessarily occur in many instances of transient myocardial ischemia.

V. CONCLUSIONS

Based on atrial pacing studies, exercise studies, hemodynamic monitoring and transient coronary artery obstruction during balloon angioplasty, it is clear that pain is the *final* event in the sequence of events that characterizes the ischemic episode. In vasospastic angina, there is first a reduction in coronary blood flow followed by hemodynamic evidence of left ventricular dysfunction and then ECG changes. In exertion-related angina, increases in the work of the heart lead to the hemodynamic abnormalities which are followed by ECG changes. Angina — when it occurs — follows the ECG changes.

REFERENCES

1. R. V. Markham, Jr., M. D. Winniford, B. G. Firth, P. Nicod, G. J. Dehmer, S. E. Lewis, and L. D. Hillis. Symptomatic, electrocardiographic, metabolic, and hemodynamic alterations during pacing-induced myocardial ischemia. *Am. J. Cardiol.*, *51*:1589 (1983).
2. M. T. Upton, S. K. Rerych, G. E. Newman, S. Port, F. R. Cobb, and R. H. Jones. Detecting abnormalities in left ventricular function during exercise before angina and ST-segment depression. *Circulation, 62*:341 (1980).
3. S. Chierchia, C. Brunelli, I. Simonetti, M. Lazzari, and A. Maseri. Sequence of events in angina at rest: Primary reduction in coronary flow. *Circulation, 61*:759 (1980).
4. U. Sigwart, M. Grbic, M. Payot, J.-J. Goy, A. Essinger, and A. Fischer. Ischemic events during coronary artery balloon occlusion. In *Silent Myocardial Ischemia* (W. Rutishauser and H. Roskamm, eds.), Springer–Verlag, Berlin, 1984, pp. 29–36.
5. A. M. Hauser, V. Gangadharan, R. G. Ramos, S. Gordon, and G. C. Timmis. Sequence of mechanical, electrocardiographic and clinical effects of repeated coronary artery occlusion in human beings: Echocardiographic observations during coronary angioplasty. *J. Am. Coll. Cardiol., 5*:193 (1985).

4

Left Ventricular Dysfunction and Myocardial Blood Flow Disturbances During Episodes of Silent Myocardial Ischemia

Is less myocardium at jeopardy than during symptomatic ischemia?

We have already discussed in Chapter 2 the possibility that altered pain perception is a cause of silent myocardial ischemia. This chapter will explore the possibility that asymptomatic ischemia is "silent" because less myocardium is ischemic compared to symptomatic episodes. In this regard, comparative studies of left ventricular function in symptomatic and asymptomatic myocardial ischemia can be categorized into two major types: (1) hemodynamic changes recorded with catheters in the right and/or left heart chambers, and (2) ventriculography performed either invasively with contrast agent, or noninvasively with radionuclide ventriculography or echocardiography.

I. HEMODYNAMIC CHANGES DURING SILENT MYOCARDIAL ISCHEMIA

One of the most comprehensive of these studies was the report by Chierchia and colleagues [1]. These investigators studied 14 patients admitted to the coronary care unit because of rest angina. Left ventricular or pulmonary pressures and systemic arterial hemodynamics were measured for a mean of 13.6 hours during continuing electrocardiographic monitoring. Eighty-four percent (or 247) of the 293 episodes of transient ST and segment and T wave changes were completely asymptomatic. Figure 1 shows a computer plot of hemodynamic variables recorded in these episodes. Most (63%) of these asymptomatic episodes were associated with an elevation in the left ventricular end-diastolic or pulmonary artery diastolic pressure of 5 mmHg or more; a smaller number (15%) had elevations of 2–4 mmHg (Table 1). In 22% there were no changes or less than a 2-mmHg rise in pressure. Peak contraction and relaxation indices using dP/dt (the first derivative of left ventricular pressure) were reduced considerably (to 100 mmHg/sec or more) in over 88% of the asymptomatic episodes. That these hemodynamic changes represented ischemia in these patients was confirmed by primary reductions in coronary sinus blood flow calculated from changes in coronary sinus oxygen saturation. Although the patients in this sereis represented examples of coronary vasospasm, not all instances of silent myocardial ischemia are due to this mechanism.

The hemodynamic changes during the 247 asymptomatic episodes were compared to those occurring during the 46 symptomatic episodes (Figure 2). The comparisons were further subdivided by type of ST segment changes (depression or elevation). It was of interest that the mean duration of the asymptomatic episodes was significantly shorter than the symptomatic episodes (253 ± 19 sec vs. 674 ± 396 sec, $p < 0.001$). Furthermore, the left ventricular end-diastolic pressure did not rise as high in the asymp-

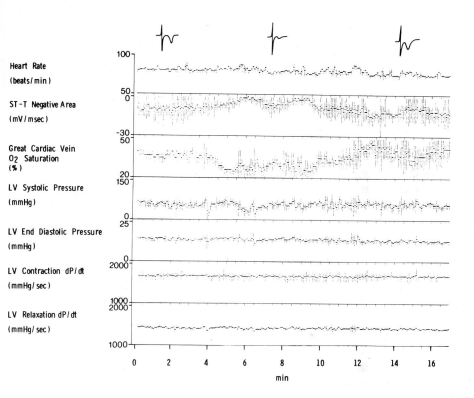

Figure 1   Computer plot of an asymptomatic episode of pseudo-normalization of an inverted T wave (decrease in ST–T negative area) in a patient with anterior ischemia. In this patient there was no increase of left ventricular (LV) end-diastolic pressure and the peak contraction and relaxation dP/dt were not altered, although there was a reduction of great cardiac vein oxygen saturation preceding and accompanying the electrocardiographic change. (From S. Chierchia, M. Lazzari, B. Freedman, C. Brunelli, and A. Maseri. *J. Am. Coll. Cardiol., 1*:924, 1983.)

Table 1 Hemodynamic Changes During Transient Asymptomatic Episodes of ST Segment or T Wave Changes

Category	Δ LVEDP or Δ PADP (mm Hg)				Δ dP/dt ⩾ 100 (mm Hg/s)			Δ LVEDP < 2 Plus Δ dP/dt C or R < 100
	n	⩾ 5	3 or 4	< 2	n	C	R	
ST↑	61	54	6	1	50	50	49	1/1
ST↓	81	43	14	24*	55	44	43	11/17
T↑	105	59	17	29	105	83	79	11/29
Total	247	156	37	54*	210	177	171	23/47

*Seven had pulmonary diastolic pressure measurements only.
Δ dP/dt C or R = change in peak left ventricular contraction or relaxation of dP/dt; Δ LVEDP or Δ PADP = change in left ventricular end-diastolic pressure or pulmonary artery diastolic pressure; ST↑ or ↓ = transient ST segment elevation or depression ⩾ 0.15 mV; T↑ = transient pseudonormalization or peaking of inverted or flat T waves.
(From S. Chierchia, M. Lazzari, B. Freedman, C. Brunelli, and A. Maseri. *J. Am. Coll. Cardiol.*, 1:924, 1983.)

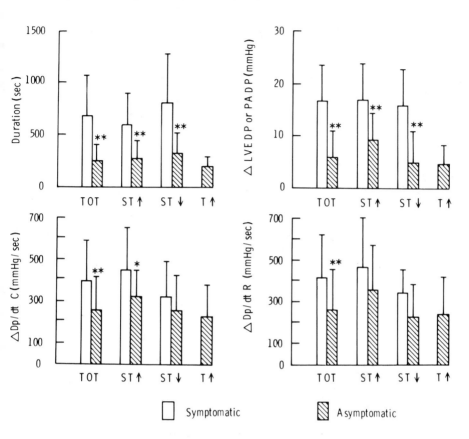

Figure 2 Comparison of symptomatic and asymptomatic episodes of ST segment and T wave changes. The mean values and standard deviation are plotted for the duration of episodes, the increases in left ventricular end-diastolic (LVEDP) (or pulmonary artery diastolic [PADP]) pressure and reductions of left ventricular peak contraction (C) and relaxation (R) dP/dt. P values for comparison of symptomatic and asymptomatic episodes: $* = < 0.01.$ $** = <$ 0.001. Overall, asymptomatic episodes were shorter and were accompanied by lesser degrees of left ventricular impairment, ST↑ or ↓ = transient ST segment elevation or depression; T↑ = transient pseudonormalization or peaking of inverted or flat T waves; TOT = total. (From S. Chierchia, M. Lazzari, B. Freedman, C. Brunelli, and A. Maseri. *J. Am. Coll. Cardiol.*, *1*:924, 1983.)

tomatic episodes (5.9 ± 5.0 mmHg vs. 16.5 ± 6.9 mmHg, p <
0.001). Using peak contraction dP/dt as an index of contractility,
the authors also reported less of an impairment in systolic function during the asymptomatic episodes (252 ± 156 mmHg/sec vs.
395 ± 199 mmHg/sec, p < 0.001). Diastolic function was characterized by peak relaxation dP/dt; again the reduction in this
measurement was less in the asymptomatic episodes (259 ± 191
mmHg/sec vs. 413 ± 209 mmHg/sec, p < 0.001). These trends
were observed regardless of the type of ST segment abnormality.
The authors concluded that in their study population, "asymptomatic episodes were usually characterized by a shorter duration
and a lesser degree of ischemic left ventricular dysfunction than
are the symptomatic episodes, although there is a considerable
degree of overlap both in the group data nad the results from individual patients." The authors speculated that asymptomatic episodes may represent lesser degrees of myocardial ischemia, though
they acknowledged that the wide overlap in duration of episodes
and degree of left ventricular impairment observed in the group
data (as well as multiple episodes in individual patients) suggest
that the severity of ischemia was not the only factor involved in
the genesis of anginal pain.

II. RADIONUCLIDE AND CONTRAST
VENTRICULOGRAPHY

Other investigators have utilized radionuclide ventriculography to
evaluate left ventricular function in asymptomatic subjects. Our
laboratory [2] employed a computerized program to calculate
regional ejection fractions at rest and during exercise. Figure 3
depicts the computer generated left ventricular regions of interest
that were evaluated in 40 patients, 16 with and 24 without silent
myocardial ischemia. The clinical and arteriographic features of
these two groups of patients were similar (Table 2) and so was
their ejection fraction response to exercise (Table 3). None of the
asymptomatic patients had pain with their test, nor were they receiving any antianginal medications that could have modified the
pain response. During exercise, global ejection fraction decreased
by 0.06 in both groups. Even when differences in resting (baseline) values were considered, the relative decreases were not significant (9% vs. 12%). Analysis of each of the three ventricular

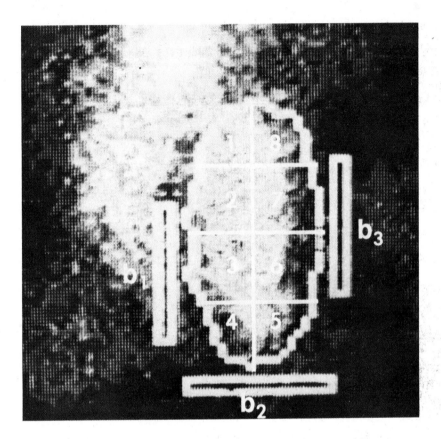

Figure 3 End-diastolic image of heart in left anterior oblique position with hand-drawn left ventricular outline. Eight regions of interest (subdivisions within the left ventricle) are indicated by the numbers 1 to 8. Regions 2 and 3 represent the anteroseptal, 4 and 5 the apical and 6 and 7 the inferoposterior regions. Regions 1 and 8 are not used in analysis of regional ejection fraction because of the overlying cardiac valves and other structures. Three background regions (rectangles b_1, b_2 and b_3 located outside the left ventricular perimeter) are considered using an automated background correction algorithm. (From P. F. Cohn, E. J. Brown, J. Wynne, B. L. Holman, and H. L. Atkins. *J. Am. Coll. Cardiol.*, *1*:931, 1983.)

Table 2   Clinical and Arteriographic Features in Patients With (Group 1) and Without (Group 2) Silent Myocardial Ischemia

	Group 1 (16 patients)	p	Group 2 (24 patients)
Age (yr)	55 ± 3[a]	NS	54 ± 2
Male	13	NS	19
Prior MI	10	NS	15
CAD			
3 vessel	7	NS	11
2 vessel	6	NS	7
1 vessel	3	NS	6

[a] = mean value ± standard error of the mean.
CAD = coronary artery disease; MI = myocardial infarctions; NS = not significant; p = probability value.
(From P. F. Cohn, E. J. Brown, J. Wynne, B. L. Holman, and H. L. Atkins. *J. Am. Coll. Cardiol.*, *1*:931, 1983).

Table 3   Radionuclide Ejection Fraction in Patients With (Group 1) and Without (Group 2) Silent Myocardial Ischemia

	Group 1 (16 patients)	p	Group 2 (24 patients)
Global			
Rest	0.60 ± 0.04	NS	0.53 ± 0.04
Exercise	0.54 ± 0.04	NS	0.47 ± 0.04
Anteroseptal region			
Rest	0.60 ± 0.04	NS	0.51 ± 0.04
Exercise	0.56 ± 0.04	NS	0.45 ± 0.04
Apical region			
Rest	0.65 ± 0.06	NS	0.57 ± 0.05
Exercise	0.62 ± 0.06	NS	0.52 ± 0.05
Inferoposterior region			
Rest	0.70 ± 0.07	NS	0.66 ± 0.05
Exercise	0.64 ± 0.04	NS	0.59 ± 0.05

NS = not significant; p = probability value.
(From P. F. Cohn, E. J. Brown, J. Wynne, B. L. Holman, and H. L. Atkins. *J. Am. Coll. Cardiol.*, *1*:931, 1983.)

regions of interest showed no significant difference in the degree of reduction during exercise. In addition, the percent of normal regions at rest, i.e., with ejection fraction >0.50, that demonstrated a decrease during exercise was 60% in both groups (19/33 vs. 22/46). We concluded that in these 40 patients — in whom the prevalence of myocardial infarction and multivessel disease was similar — no discernible differences in wall motion abnormalities or ejection fraction were found.

Iskandrian and Hakki [3] approached this problem in a slightly different manner. They compared left ventricular function during exercise radionuclide ventriculography in anginal patients who either did or did not have their usual angina during the exercise procedure. Thirty-one patients had angina during the test and 43 did not. Multivessel disease was present in equal percentages in both groups of patients, as were a variety of clinical factors. Although the global ejection fraction was similar at rest in both groups, it fell to a greater extent in the symptomatic group (-0.045 ± 0.076 vs. -0.01 ± 0.094, $p < 0.01$). Other measurements (wall motion score, end-systolic volume, etc.) showed similar trends (Figures 4 and 5). Only about half of the patients in each group had ischemic ST depression during their tests (Table 4).

The authors concluded that even though asymptomatic myocardial ischemia may occur in patients with extensive coronary artery disease and be associated with abnormal exercise left ventricular function, in general patients with symptomatic episodes have worse exercise left ventricular function than those with asymptomatic episodes.

Ratib and colleagues [4] performed isotope ventriculography in 25 patients who did not develop chest pain during exercise and found no differences in left ventricular function when compared to 14 patients who did develop angina with exercise (Figure 6). These results are similar to those from our laboratory, as opposed to those of Iskandrian and Hakki. The phase analysis techniques used in this study are different from those of regional ejection fraction analysis, but the results are equally valid.

Gleichmann and colleagues [5] studied wall motion disorders during contrast ventriculography with bicycle exercise in 141 patients with coronary artery disease. Four combinations were used: angina with wall motion disorders; angina without wall motion disorders; no angina with wall motion disorders; and neither angina

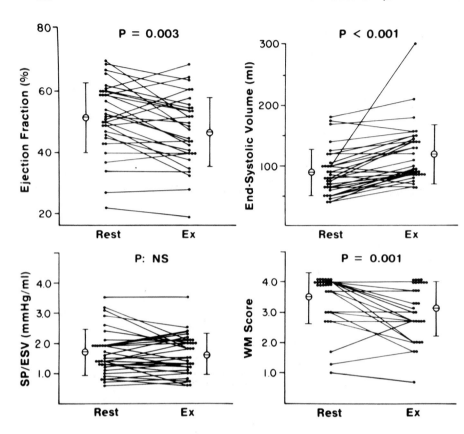

Figure 4   Left ventricular ejection fraction, end-systolic volume, systolic blood pressure-end systolic volume ratio (SP/ESV) and wall motion (WM) score at rest and during exercise (Ex) in patients with angina during the test. The means and standard deviations are also shown. NS = not significant. (From A. S. Iskandrian and A–H. Hakki. *Am. J. Cardiol.*, *53*:1239, 1984.)

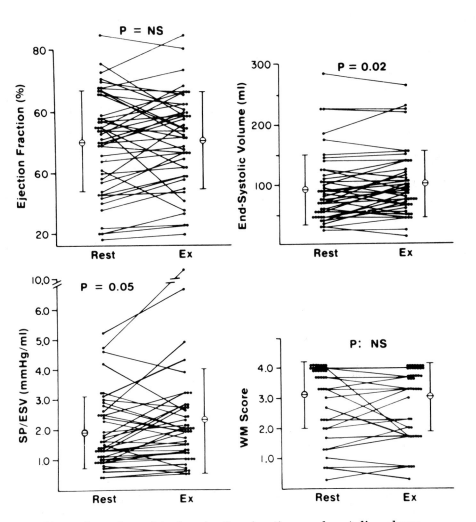

Figure 5   Left ventricular ejection fraction, end-systolic volume, systolic blood pressure-end-systolic volume ratio (SP/ESV) and wall motion (WM) score at rest and during exercise in patients without angina. NS = not significant. (From A. S. Iskandrian and A-H. Hakki. *Am. J. Cardiol.*, 53:1239, 1984.)

Table 4   Left Ventricular Function During Exercise in Relation to
Ejection Fraction at Rest and During Exercise — Electrocardiographic Changes

| | Positive Ex ECG | |
LVEF	Group I	Group II
≥ 50% at rest, ab response to Ex	5/15	8/16
≥ 50% at rest, NL response to Ex	1/4	2/9
< 50% at rest, ab response to Ex	9/12	3/9
< 50% at rest, NL response to Ex	0/15	4/9
Total	15/31	17/43

ab = abnormal (failure to increase EF by ≥ 5% from rest to exercise); Ex =
exercise; LVEF = left ventricular ejection fraction; NL = normal. Group I =
angina. Group II = no angina.
(From A. S. Iskandrian and A-H Hakki. *Am. J. Cardiol.*, *53*:1239, 1984.)

nor wall motion disorders. About 25% of patients fell into each of
the groups. Thus, the presence of angina could not clearly differ-
entiate normal and abnormal left ventricular function with exercise. For example, more than 50% of the patients with one-vessel
disease and no prior infarction had no angina but had hypokinesis
or akinesis. This combination was less frequent in patients with
two-vessel disease (3%) or three-vessel disease (25%). The four
possible combinations are depicted in Figure 7 and a typical
example depicted in Figure 8. The severe nature of these silent
episodes was further confirmed by the rise in left ventricular end-
diastolic pressure during exercise in many of the patients with wall
motion disorders. However, the higher prevalence of one-vessel
disease does suggest less myocardium at jeopardy.

III. MYOCARDIAL BLOOD FLOW STUDIES

Myocardial blood flow (perfusion) studies are generally of two
types: quantitative and invasive vs. qualitative and noninvasive.
A prime example of the former type is the xenon-133 clearance
technique for measuring regional myocardial blood flow. Because
of physiologic restraints, this technique has been shown in several
centers around the world to be most reliable when the same patient

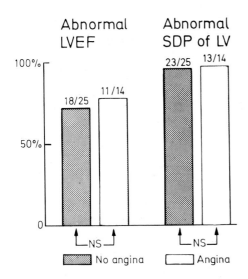

Figure 6   The numbers of patients with an abnormal response of left ventricular (LV) function during exercise. A failure to increase left ventricular ejection fraction (LVEF) by 5% or more was considered abnormal. Using this criterion, 72% of the patients without angina and 78% of the patients with angina had an abnormal LVEF during exercise. The authors established the upper limit of normal for standard deviation of peak (SDP) of LV as 14°, which is the mean plus two standard deviations measured in ten normals at maximum exercise. There was no statistical difference between the two groups. SDP is an index of the degree of synchronicity of LV wall motion. (From O. Ratib, A. Righetti, and W. Rutishauser. In *Silent Myocardial Ischemia* [W. Rutishauser and H. Roskamm, eds.], Springer–Verlag, Berlin, 1984, pp. 84–89.)

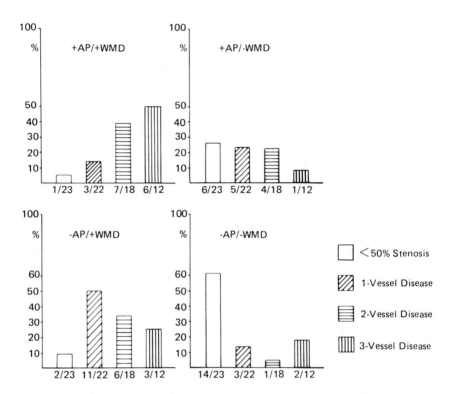

Figure 7   Left ventricular exercise angiography: frequency of angina pectoris (AP) and wall motion disorders (WMD) in 75 patients with coronary artery disease (CAD) without scar. (From U. Gleichmann, D. FaBbender, H. Mannebach, J. Vogt, and G. Trieb. In *Silent Myocardial Ischemia* [W. Rutishauser and H. Roskamm, eds.], Springer–Verlag, Berlin, 1984, pp. 71–77.)

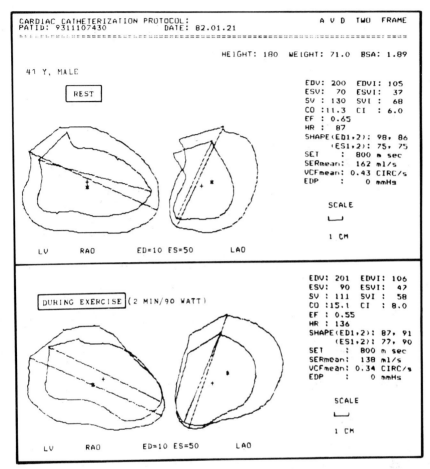

Figure 8   Computerized global left ventricular volume analysis at rest (top) and with exercise (bottom) in a patient with 75% left anterior descending stenosis and no angina pectoris, but significant akinesis with a drop in ejection fraction from 65% at rest to 55% with exercise. (From U. Gleichmann, D. FaBbender, H. Mannebach, J. Vogt, and G. Trieb. In *Silent Myocardial Ischemia* [W. Rutishauser and H. Roskamm, eds.], Springer-Verlag, Berlin, 1984, pp. 71–77.)

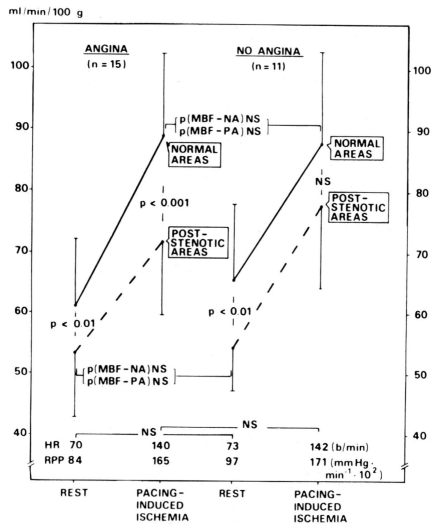

Figure 9 Regional myocardial blood flow (MBF) at rest and during rapid atrial pacing in 15 patients with and 11 patients without angina pectoris during ischemia. NA = normal areas; PA = post-stenotic areas; HR = heart rate; RPP = rate-pressure product. (From W. G. Daniel, H–J. Engel, H. Hundeshage, and P. R. Lichtlen. In *Silent Myocardial Ischemia* [W. Rutishauser and H. Roskamm, eds.], Springer–Verlag, Berlin, 1984, pp. 45–49.)

is used as his or her own control. One of the pioneers in this work
is Lichtlen. Recently he and his colleagues reported their results
in 11 patients with coronary artery disease not experiencing angina
during ischemia induced by rapid atrial pacing [6]. Fifteen patients had angina during these studies and served as a control group.
Figure 9 depicts the results: blood flow increased in poststenotic
areas much less than in normal regions during rapid atrial pacing,
but no differences were found between the angina and nonangina
groups. However, individual responses did show a tendency for
flow to be actually reduced in some patients with angina (Figure
10). The reason for this is not clear, but a vasospastic mechanism
may be implicated.

The prime example of a qualitative, noninvasive method for evaluating myocardial perfusion is the thallium-201 scintigram. Righetti
and colleagues [7] found that coronary patients showing perfusion
defects without angina had a smaller number of ischemic segments
despite a higher double product; Table 5 depicts the clinical and angiographic features of the two groups. By contrast, Reisman et al. [8]
found similar amounts of thallium perfusion defects in their patients.

Hinrich and colleagues [9] correlated results of lactate extraction and thallium scintigraphy in 9 asymptomatic patients with
angiographically proven coronary artery disease. In 3 patients, no
myocardial lactate production at rest or after atrial pacing was
observed and thallium scintigraphy was normal (an example is
depicted in Figure 11a–c). In 6 others, patients had both significant defects and lactate production (Figure 12a–c). Coronary
sinus blood flow increased to the same degree in both groups of
patients. The authors concluded that the absence of metabolic
and perfusion abnormalities probably indicated less myocardium
at jeopardy, despite the same degree of ST segment depression
during atrial pacing or exercise ECG.

Another type of myocardial perfusion technique utilizes an
intravenous infusion of rubidium-82. Positrontomograms of rubidium uptake were made for five regions of interest by Deanfield et
al. [10] during 24-hour ambulatory monitoring, exercise tests
and cold pressor tests in 34 patients with histories of angina. An
example of the ECG and perfusion abnormalities with and without angina is depicted in Figure 13. There was no significant difference in the change in uptake of rubidium–82 in the abnormal
segment of myocardium between exercise tests accompanied by

ml/min/100 g

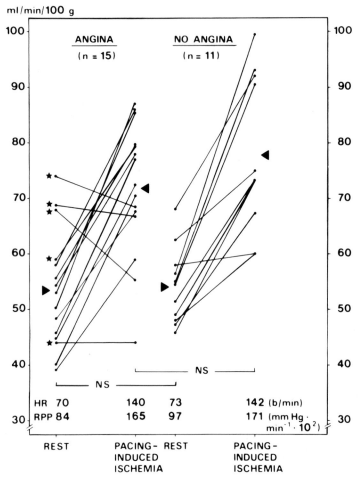

Figure 10   Regional myocardial blood flow in poststenotic areas
of 15 patients with and 11 patients without angina pectoris during
rapid atrial pacing-induced ischemia.   ★ = severe angina. (From
W. G. Daniel, H-J. Engel, H. Hundeshage, and P. R. Lichtlen. In
Silent Myocardial Ischemia [W. Rutishauser and H. Roskamm,
eds.], Springer-Verlag, Berlin, pp. 45-49.)

Table 5 Comparison of Multiple Parameters, Between Coronary Patients With and Without Angina, in the Group of Patients Showing Signs of Ischemia on ECG and on Tl-201 Images

	Ischemia on ECG		Ischemia on Tl-201 scintigraphy	
	Angina ($n = 90$)	No Angina ($n = 77$)	Angina ($n = 111$)	No Angina ($n = 143$)
Age (years)	51 ± 1	54 ± 1	54 ± 1	52 ± 1
Males	81	72	101	134
Hx of angina	69	57	80	81
Hx of MI	33	44[a]	48	80[b]
MI on ECG	22	32[a]	31	65[b]
Beta-blockers	51	36	63	71
Digitalis	77	8	11	19
Double product ($mmHg\ min^{-1}$) 10^2	196 ± 6	232 ± 5^{b}	196 ± 5	225 ± 4^{b}
One vessel	40	33	49	73
Two vessels	30	27	37	47
Three vessels	20	17	25	23
LAD	60	55	74	92
CX	45	42	55	70
RC	55	41	69	74
LVEF (%)	60 ± 1	60 ± 1	59 ± 1	58 ± 1
Mean of ischemic segments (Tl-201)	$2.3 \pm 0.1^{*}$	1.9 ± 0.1	$2.3 \pm 0.1^{*}$	2.0 ± 0.1

$^{a}p < 0.05$. $^{b}p < 0.01$. Hx - history; MI - myocardial infarction; LAD - left anterior descending; CX - circumflex; RC - right coronary; LVEF - left ventricular ejection fraction

(From A. Righetti, O. Ratib, B. El-Harake, and W. Rutishauser. In *Silent Myocardial Ischemia* (W. Rutishauser and H. Roskamm, eds.), Springer-Verlag, Berlin, 1984, pp. 50-57.)

A   H.B., ♂, 57 yr.

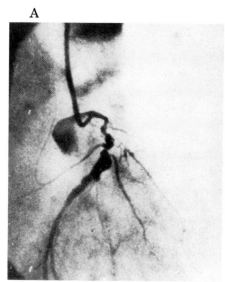 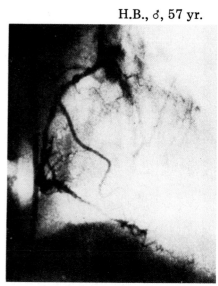

B   H.B., ♂, 57 yr.

Rest   Exercise   Pacing

I		V₁

17% ◄——————Lactate extraction rate——————► -39%

C H.B., ♂, 57 yr.

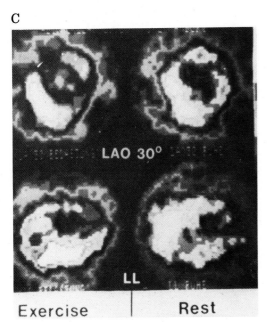

Figure 11 A-C   Asymptomatic patient with a severe left anterior descending (LAD) stenosis (A) accompanied by ST-segment depression but without lactate production (B) or thallium defects (C) during exercise or atrial pacing. LAO = left anterior oblique view; LL = left lateral view. (From A. Hinrichs, W. Kupper, C. L. V. Hamm, and W. Bleifeld. In *Silent Myocardial Ischemia* [W. Rutishauser and H. Roskamm, eds.], Springer-Verlag, Berlin, 1984, pp. 50–57.)

A   R.S., ♀, 43 yr.

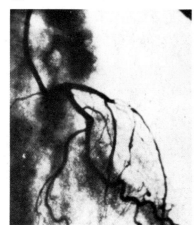
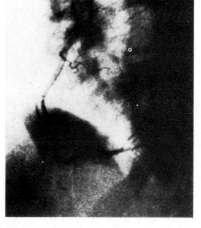

B   R.S., ♀, 43 yr.

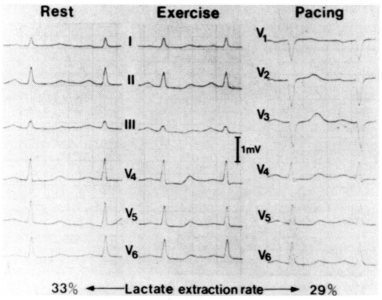

C   R.S., ♀, 43 yr.

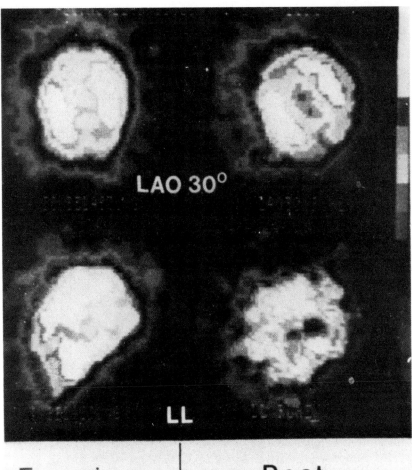

Figure 12 A–C   Asymptomatic patient with severe left anterior descending (LAD) stenoses (A) corresponding to ST-segment depression and myocardial lactate production (B), and a reversible thallium defect of the left ventricular anterior wall (C) during exercise or atrial pacing.   LAO = left anterior oblique view; LL = left lateral view.   (From A. Hinrichs, W. Kupper, C. L. V. Hamm, and W. Bleifeld.   In *Silent Myocardial Ischemia* [W. Rutishauser and H. Roskamm, eds.], Springer–Verlag, Berlin, 1984, pp. 50–57.)

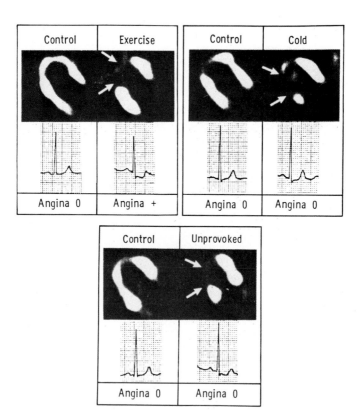

Figure 13   The tomographic slices for a single patient through the midleft ventricle showing the regional myocardial uptake of rubidium–82 in the posterior wall (PW), free wall (FW), anterior wall (a) and interventricular septum (S_1 and S_2) of the left ventricle. This demonstrates the distribution of regional perfusion during control, cold pressor, unprovoked ST depression and exercise. Evidence of regional ischemia occurred during all three tests and supported the ST segment changes as evidence of ischemia whether or not chest pain occurred. (From J. E. Deanfield, P. Ribiero, K. Oakley, S. Krikler, and A. P. Selwyn. *Am. J. Cardiol.*, *54*:1195, 1984.)

PATIENT NO. 9

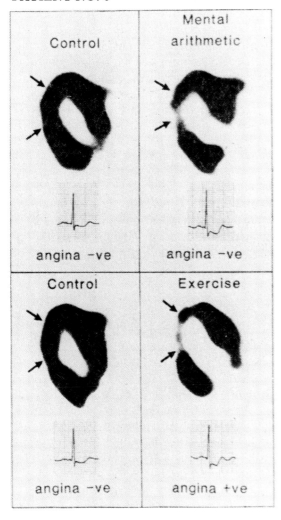

Figure 14   Changes in regional myocardial uptake of rubidium–82, and in ECG in relation to chest pain before and after mental arithmetic or exercise.   Control scans show homogeneous regional cation uptake.   Patient No. 9 shows anterior and free-wall ischaemia and ST-segment depression with mental arithmetic and exercise, but angina only after exercise (−ve = negative; +ve = positive).   (From J. E. Deanfield, M. Kensett, R. A. Wilson, M. Shea, P. Horlock, C. M. deLandsheere, and A. P. Selwyn. *Lancet*, 2:1001, 1984.)

angina and those without pain (uptake changed from 47 ± 9.8 to 38 ± 10.6 for episodes of ST segment depression with angina versus 52 ± 13 to 44 ± 12 for episodes of painless ST depression). Similarly, regional uptake changes in the abnormal segment of myocardium during unprovoked episodes of ST depression with angina were not significantly different from those found during painless episodes (from 48 ± 8.5 to 36 ± 6.6 for episodes of ST segment depression with angina versus 48 ± 7 to 37.5 ± 8.3 for episodes of painless ST depression. The same group has also documented silent myocardial ischemia during metal arithmetic [11] (Figure 14) and smoking [12].

IV. CONCLUSIONS

Despite a surprisingly large number of studies evaluating hemodynamic, ventriculographic and myocardial blood flow changes during silent myocardial ischemia, there is not consensus whether less myocardium is at jeopardy during these episodes compared to symptomatic ones.

REFERENCES

1. S. Chierchia, M. Lazzari, B. Freedman, C. Brunelli, and A. Maseri. Impairment of myocardial perfusion and function during painless myocardial ischemia. *J. Am. Coll. Cardiol.*, *1*:924 (1983).
2. P. F. Cohn, E. J. Brown, J. Wynne, B. L. Holman, and H. L. Atkins. Global and regional left ventricular ejection fraction abnormalities during exercise in patients with silent myocardial ischemia. *J. Am. Coll. Cardiol.*, *1*:931 (1983).
3. A. S. Iskandrian and A-H. Hakki. Left ventricular function in patients with coronary heart disease in the presence or absence of angina pectoris during exercise radionuclide ventriculography. *Am. J. Cardiol.*, *53*:1239 (1984).
4. O. Ratib, A. Righetti, and W. Rutishauser. Isotope ventriculography during asymptomatic ischemia. In *Silent Myocardial Ischemia* (W. Rutishauser and H. Roskamm, eds.), Springer–Verlag, Berlin, 1984, pp. 84–89.
5. U. Gleichmann, D. FaBbender, H. Mannebach, J. Vogt, and G. Trieb. Contrast ventriculography: Wall motion disorder without angina pectoris during exercise-induced ischemia. In

Silent Myocardial Ischemia (W. Rutishauser and H. Roskamm, eds.), Springer-Verlag, Berlin, 1984, pp. 71–77.

6. W. G. Daniel, H-J. Engel, H. Hundeshage, and P. R. Lichtlen. Regional myocardial blood flow under rapid atrial pacing in patients with ST-segment depression without angina pain. In *Silent Myocardial Ischemia* (W. Rutishauser and H. Roskamm, eds.), Springer-Verlag, Berlin, 1984, pp. 45–49.

7. A. Righetti, O. Ratib, B. El-Harake, and W. Rutishauser. Thallium-201 myocardial scintigraphy and electrographic findings in asymptomatic coronary patients during exercise testing. In *Silent Myocardial Ischemia* (W. Rutishauser and H. Roskamm, eds.), Springer-Verlag, Berlin, 1984, pp. 79–83.

8. S. Reisman, D. S. Berman, J. Maddahi, and H. J. C. Swan. Silent myocardial ischemia during treadmill exercise. Thallium scintigraphic and angiographic correlates (abstr). *J. Am. Coll. Cardiol.*, 5:406 (1985).

9. A. Hinrichs, W. Kupper, C. L. V. Hamm, and W. Bleifeld. Detection of silent myocardial ischemia in correlation to hemodynamic and metabolic data. In *Silent Myocardial Ischemia* (W. Rutihauser and H. Roskamm, eds.), Springer-Verlag, Berlin, 1984, pp. 50–57.

10. J. E. Deanfield, M. Shea, P. Ribiero, C. M. deLandsheere, R. A. Wilson, P. Horlock, and A. P. Selwyn. Transient ST segment depression as a marker of myocardial ischemia during daily life: A physiological validation in patients with angina and coronary disease. *Am. J. Cardiol.*, 54:1195 (1984).

11. J. E. Deanfield, M. Kensett, R. A. Wilson, M. Shea, P. Horlock, C. M. deLandsheere, and A. P. Selwyn. Silent myocardial ischemia due to mental stress. *Lancet*, 2:1001 (1984).

12. J. E. Deanfield, M. T. Shea, R. Wilson, C. M. deLandsheere, A. Jonathan, and A. P. Selwyn. Direct effect of smoking causes silent ischemia in patients with angina pectoris (abstr). *J. Am. Coll. Cardiol.*, 5:506, 1985.

II

PREVALENCE OF ASYMPTOMATIC CORONARY ARTERY DISEASE

5

Prevalence of Silent Myocardial Ischemia

Is the presence of pain in persons with coronary artery disease just the "tip of the iceberg"? Are most of these persons actually free of pain all of the time or most of the time? These are intriguing,

71

Table 1   Prevalence of Coronary Artery Stenosis at Autopsy

	Men		Women	
Age (yr)	Proportion affected	Pooled mean ± SEP[a] (%)	Proportion affected	Pooled mean ± SEP (%)
30–39	57/2,954	1.9 ± 0.3	5/1,545	0.3 ± 0.1
40–49	234/4,407	5.5 ± 0.3	18/1,778	1.0 ± 0.2
50–59	488/5,011	9.7 ± 0.4	62/1,934	3.2 ± 0.4
60–69	569/4,641	12.3 ± 0.5	130/1,726	7.5 ± 0.6
Totals	1,348/17,013		215/6,983	
Population-weighted mean[b]		6.4 ± 0.2		2.6 ± 0.2

[a]Standard error of the per cent.
[b]Population weighting was performed by use of the 1970 U.S. Census figures.
(From G. A. Diamond and J. S. Forrester. *N. Engl. J. Med., 300*:1350, 1979.)

but unresolved, questions. They will be addressed in four distinct areas in this chapter.

I. SILENT MYOCARDIAL ISCHEMIA IN PERSONS WITH TOTALLY ASYMPTOMATIC CORONARY ARTERY DISEASE

This is an extremely difficult area to obtain "hard data" in. How are persons who are free of symptoms to be convinced of the need to undergo coronary arteriography in order to confirm the diagnosis of asymptomatic coronary artery disease? It is true that fortuitous — and anecdotal — "case finding" in this syndrome occurs commonly enough to draw attention to the problem, but systematic surveys are rare. This is because of concerns raised about subjecting asymptomatic individuals to an invasive procedure with a small but definite morbidity and mortality. For example, mortality as a result of cardiac catheterization and angiography can range from 0–1% in different centers.

Another approach to estimating the prevalence of asymptomatic disease is through pathologic surveys of atherosclerotic heart disease in adult populations who were apparently free of clinical coronary artery disease at time of death, and died of trauma or noncardiac causes. Diamond and Forester conducted the most comprehensive review in 1979 [1]. They summarized their data in

Table 1, which breaks down the autopsy studies by age and sex. In the nearly 24,000 persons studied, the mean prevalence of coronary artery disease was 4.5%. The population-weighted mean (obtained by use of the 1970 U.S. Census figures) was 6.4 ± 0.2% for men aged 30–69 and 2.6 ± 0.2% for women aged 30–69. This percentage increased with increasing age. Since these figures are obtained from autopsy data, they may overestimate the true incidence of this syndrome for two reasons. First, unless the autopsy procedure employs techniques for injecting the coronary arteries, the "collapsed" lumen examined by the pathologist may exaggerate the luminal narrowing caused by a given lesion during life. Second, even when the degree of narrowing is as it was during life, there is no certainty that lesions in the 50–60% category were hemodynamically significant when the person was alive. In other words, not all asymptomatic coronary artery disease present at autopsy is necessarily ischemia-producing coronary artery disease. Just as those lesions were not hemodynamically significant, others may represent "end-stage" or "burnt-out" stages of the disease process: arteries became occluded, infarctions occurred, scar tissue formed, but there is no longer evidence of active ischemia.

Another approach to estimating the prevalence of coronary artery disease in asymptomatic persons is by reviewing coronary angiographic data. In their report, Diamond and Forrester [1] did that type of analysis, as well. The data that they found suggested that the prevalence of coronary artery disease in asymptomatic adults was about 4%. These patients had undergone cardiac catheterization for reasons other than chest pain (evaluation of valvular heart disease, abnormal ECGs, etc.). Since these catheterization laboratory figures reflect a skewered population in that they were selected to undergo the procedure, one might argue that the 4% figure is too low. Perhaps an "average" of the autopsy and angiographic figures (about 5%) would be more useful. However, in neither the autopsy review or the angiographic review are data supplied about the prevalence of active ischemia in these asymptomatic subjects.

Screening large numbers of asymptomatic persons with exercise tests and *then* subjecting positive responders to coronary angiography is a useful technique for estimating the number of individuals with *both* asymptomatic disease and active ischemia. Several such studies have been reported. In one small study, investigators at Yale University [2] exercised 129 workers in a nearby industrial plant. Sixteen subjects had an abnormal exercise test and 13 of these also had coronary artery calcification on fluorscopy. The 13 men underwent coronary arteriography; 12 had at least 50% stenosis in one coronary artery. Thus, 12 of the anginal 129 subjects, or about 9%, had both asymptomatic coronary artery disease and silent myocardial ischemia. U.S. Air Force studies in 1390 men revealed 111 with positive exercise tests in a single lead, of which 34 (or about 2.5%) had 50% or greater lesions [3]. The mean age of these patients was 43 years; all were males.

In Norway, Erickssen et al. [4] studied 2014 male office workers who were aged 40–59 years (mean age 50). Sixty-nine had at least 50% stenosis in one coronary artery and 50 of these (or 2.8% of the total) were completely asymptomatic. This percentage is very similar to that of the U.S. Air Force study. These figures must be considered as conservative estimates, since it is possible that some asymptomatic individuals did not manifest silent ischemia on the one screening exercise test and, therefore, were not selected for coronary angiographic studies. Furthermore, exercise tests in general have a certain percentage of false-negative tests, whereas coronary angiography tends to underestimate the severity of lesions. Thus, the figure of 5% cited earlier for the prevalence of asymptomatic anatomic disease probably exaggerates only slightly the true prevalence of hemodynamically significant asymptomatic disease, i.e., disease capable of producing ischemia during physiological stress.

II. SILENT MYOCARDIAL ISCHEMIA IN INDIVIDUALS ASYMPTOMATIC AFTER A MYOCARDIAL INFARCTION

It has been estimated that 500,000 patients recover from myocardial infarctions annually. Of these, 30–40% have their courses complicated by persistent angina, heart failure or serious arrhythmias [5]. The rest are asymptomatic at time of discharge. Of these 300,000 or so latter individuals, about one-third (100,000) have evidence of ischemia on postinfarction exercise tests [6–8] and half of these patients have no symptoms with their ischemia. Thus, about 50,000 asymptomatic postinfarction patients per year have silent myocardial ischemia in the initial 30-day postinfarction period.

III. SILENT MYOCARDIAL ISCHEMIA IN PATIENTS WITH ANGINA

The number of patients with angina who also have asymptomatic episodes of myocardial ischemia is large, but the exact percentage is unknown. About 3–4 million patients per year are seen by physicians because of anginal complaints. When I reviewed the literature on positive exercise tests, lactate determinations, abnormal ventriculograms, etc. in those studies that reported symptoms, I found that about a third of symptomatic patients (Table 2) had at least one documented episode of silent myocardial ischemia [9]. The figure is higher when ST depression on Holter monitoring is considered. Based on studies by Deanfield and colleagues [10] and by Fazzini and colleagues [11], the number of patients with silent ischemia on Holter monitoring can range from 60 to 100% of the study population. Furthermore, the silent episodes outnumber the painful ones at least three or four to one. This is discussed later in Chapter 8.

IV. SUDDEN DEATH AND MYOCARDIAL INFARCTION IN PATIENTS WITHOUT PRIOR HISTORIES OF ANGINA

Although this is an "indirect" way of estimating the population with asymptomatic coronary artery disease, it provides important data. Presumably, individuals who die suddenly or experience a myocardial infarction as their initial manifestation of coronary artery disease and who have extensive coronary atherosclerosis at autopsy or coronary angiography did not develop those lesions overnight. Much of the disease must have been present, silent and undetected, for weeks, months or even years prior to the actual event. This is the natural history — amply documented — of coronary atherosclerosis. That the precipitating event, such as rupture of a plaque into a vessel lumen, could have been sudden is not in dispute, but the atherosclerotic substrate took months and years to develop. With that in mind, it is important to note that one-quarter to one-half (depending on the series) of the 300,000 individuals who die suddenly each year with coronary artery disease found at autopsy had no prior cardiac history [12, 13]. As Kuller [13] has written, "The large pool of individuals currently over the age of 30 or 40 with silent but significant coronary

Table 2 Myocardial Ischemia Without Anginal Symptoms

Abnormality Suggestive of Myocardial Ischemia	Patients With CAD Manifesting Abnormality		
	Total group (n)	Group With Angina[a]	
		no.	%
Abnormal left ventricular wall motion	87	33	39%
Pacing contrast ventriculogram[1]	8	3	38%
Pacing contrast ventriculogram[2]	8	6	75%
Exercise radionuclide ventriculogram[5]	63	18	29%
Exercise radionuclide ventriculogram[6]	8	6	75%
Abnormal lactate metabolism	36	9	25%
Pacing study[7]	14	1	7%
Pacing study[8]	22	8	36%
Abnormal myocardial perfusion scintigrams	64	26	40%
Thallium-201 study[9]	35	20	57%
Rubidium-81 study[10]	29	6	19%
Electrocardiographic stress test	568	186	32%
Treadmill test[11]	135	23	17%
Treadmill test[12]	122	32	26%
Bicycle and two-step test[13]	59	15	26%
Treadmill test[14]	146	68	45%
Treadmill test[15]	102	48	47%
Total	755	254	34%

[a] Although not symptomatic during this test, almost all patients in these studies had a history of angina or prior myocardial infarction (see text).
CAD = coronary artery disease.
(From P. F. Cohn. Am. J. Cardiol, 45:697, 1980. Numbers in superscript refer to studies cited in this article.)

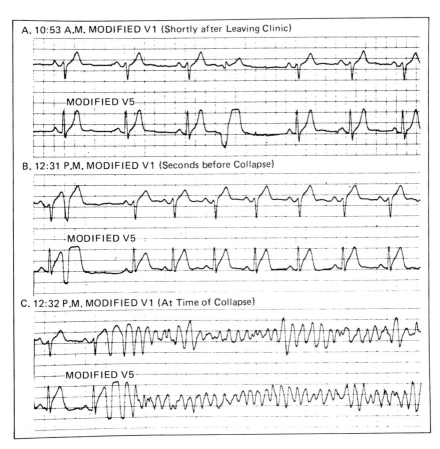

A. 10:53 A.M. MODIFIED V1 (Shortly after Leaving Clinic)

MODIFIED V5

B. 12:31 P.M. MODIFIED V1 (Seconds before Collapse)

MODIFIED V5

C. 12:32 P.M. MODIFIED V1 (At Time of Collapse)

MODIFIED V5

Figure 1 (A) The subject's first ventricular premature depolarization, which was detected approximately a half hour after he left the clinic. No significant changes in the S–T segment were noted at the time of this late-cycle premature depolarization. (B) The second form of ventricular premature depolarization, which was uniformly early-cycle and associated with increased S–T segment elevation and convex S–T segment morphology. (C) The electrocardiogram at the instant of the subject's collapse. The same early-cycle ventricular premature form detected earlier initiated a four-beat run of ventricular tachycardia, which rapidly degenerated to ventricular flutter-fibrillation. (From D. D. Savage, W. P. Castelli, S. J. Anderson, and W. B. Kannel. *Am. J. Med.*, 74:148, 1983.)

atherosclerosis and stenoses will contribute to a high incidence of sudden death, at least for the next 20 or 30 years." Savage et al. [14] provide a graphic example of death in one such individual recorded on an ambulatory monitor that was performed fortuitiously as part of a Framingham study protocol (Figure 1).

Nearly half of the patients presenting with their first myocardial infarctions have not had angina beforehand [15]. Midwall and colleagues [16] noted that in general, these patients were more likely to be younger, female and have a greater prevalence of one-vessel disease (Table 3). Do they, therefore, represent a unique subset of coronary artery disease? In a study from our hospital [17], we studied 43 consecutive patients presenting with their initial myocardial infarction; 23 had no history of angina prior to the infarction, whereas 20 did. The two groups did not differ in age, smoking history, diabetes, hypertension or cholesterol levels. The prevalence of Q and non-Q wave infarcts was similar, but there was a trend toward more inferior infarctions in the asymptomatic group (65% vs. 47%) and more single-vessel disease (40% vs. 11%). Multivessel coronary artery disease is frequent enough, however, in patients without prior angina to suggest that an infarction without prior angina does not necessarily indicate less advanced coronary artery disease and, therefore, should not be considered a unique subset of coronary artery disease.

Table 3   Catheterization Data in Myocardial Infarction Patients

Parameter	Group 1 No prior AP	Group 2 AP prior to MI	Sig
Mean EDP (mm Hg)	15.8 ± 6.9	14.5 ± 6.5	NS
Mean LVEF (%)	58.7 ± 14.7	58.5 ± 14.8	NS
Collaterals	46%	71%	$p < 0.05$
One-vessel disease	38/63 (60%)	3/34 (9%)	$p < 0.005$
Two-vessel disease	18/63 (29%)	18/34 (53%)	$p < 0.05$
Three-vessel disease	7/63 (11%)	13/34 (38%)	$p < 0.005$

Abbreviations: AP, angina pectoris; Sig, significance; MI, myocardial infarction; EDP, end-diastolic pressure; LVEF, left ventricular ejection fraction; NS, not significant.
(From J. Midwall, J. Ambrose, A. Pichard, Z. Abedin, and M. V. Herman. *Chest, 81*:6, 1982.)

V. CONCLUSIONS

Silent myocardial ischemia is a ubiquitous phenomenon, present in about 5% of the asymptomatic population, about one-third of uncomplicated asymptomatic postinfarction patients and in most patients with angina. The scope of the problem is further indicated — albeit indirectly — by the large number of individuals dying suddenly or experiencing an infarction without a prior anginal history.

REFERENCES

1. G. A. Diamond and J. S. Forrester. Analysis of probability as an aid in the clinical diagnosis of coronary artery disease. *N. Engl. J. Med., 300*:1350 (1979).
2. R. A. Langou, E. K. Huang, M. J. Kelley, and L. S. Cohen. Predictive accuracy of coronary artery calcification and abnormal exercise test for coronary artery disease in asymptomatic men. *Circulation, 62*:1196 (1980).
3. V. F. Froelicher, A. J. Thompson, M. R. Longo, Jr., J. H. Triebwasser, and M. C. Lancaster. Value of exercise testing for screening asymptomatic men for latent coronary artery disease. *Prog. Cardiovasc. Dis., 16*:265 (1976).
4. J. Erikssen, I. Enge, K. Forfang, and O. Storstein. False positive diagnostic test and coronary angiographic findings in 105 presumably healthy males. *Circulation, 54*:371 (1976).
5. S. E. Epstein, S. T. Palmeri, and R. E. Patterson. Evaluation of patients after acute myocardial infarction. *N. Engl. J. Med., 307*:1487 (1982).
6. P. Theroux, D. D. Waters, C. Halphen, J-C. Debaisieux, and H. F. Mizgala. Prognostic value of exercise testing soon after myocardial infarction. *N. Engl. J. Med., 301*:341 (1979).
7. D. H. Miller and J. S. Borer. Exercise testing early after myocardial infarction: risks and benefits. *Am. J. Med., 72*:427 (1982).
8. D. M. Davidson and R. F. DeBusk. Prognostic value of a single exercise test 3 weeks after uncomplicated myocardial infarction. *Circulation, 61*:236 (1980).
9. P. F. Cohn. Silent myocardial ischemia in patients with a defective anginal warning system. *Am. J. Cardiol., 45*:697 (1980).

10. J. E. Deanfield, A. P. Selwyn, S. Chierchia, A. Maseri, P. Ribeiro, S. Krikler, and M. Morgan. Myocardial ischemia during daily life in patients with stable angina: its relations to symptoms and heart rate changes. *Lancet, 1*:753 (1983).

11. A. C. Cecchi, E. V. Dovellini, F. Marchi, P. Pucci, G. M. Santoro, and P. F. Fazzini. Silent myocardial ischemia during ambulatory electrocardiographic monitoring in patients with effort angina. *J. Am. Coll. Cardiol., 1*:934 (1983).

12. B. Lown. Sudden cardiac death: The major challenge confronting contemporary cardiology. *Am. J. Cardiol., 43*:313 (1979).

13. L. H. Kuller. Sudden death — Definition and epidemiologic considerations. *Prog. Cardiovasc. Dis., 23*:1 (1980).

14. D. D. Savage, W. P. Castelli, S. J. Anderson, and W. B. Kannel. Sudden unexpected death during ambulatory electrocardiographic monitoring: The Framingham study. *Am. J. Med., 74*:148 (1983).

15. R. W. Harper, G. Kennedy, R. W. DeSanctis, and A. M. Hutter. The incidence and pattern of angina prior to acute myocardial infarction: A study of 577 cases. *Am. Heart J., 97*:178 (1979).

16. J. Midwall, J. Ambrose, A. Pichard, Z. Abedin, and M. V. Herman. Angina pectoris before and after infarction: Angiographic correlations. *Chest, 81*:6 (1982).

17. S. A. Samuel and P. F. Cohn. Myocardial infarction without a prior history of angina pectoris: A unique subset of coronary artery disease? (abstr) *Clin. Res., 33*:224A (1985).

6
Prevalence and Distinguishing Features of Silent Myocardial Infarctions

I.   Electrocardiographic Studies
II. Autopsy Studies
III. Mechanisms to Explain the Absence of Pain. Is Diabetes
     Mellitus a Factor?
IV. Conclusions
     References

The subject of silent (unrecognized) myocardial infarction has
intrigued physicians for over 70 years. Herrick was aware of it in
his landmark paper published in 1912 [1] and anecdotal reports
throughout the 1930s and 1940s maintained interest in this seem-
ing paradox [2-5]. In 1954, Roseman reviewed the literature

and analyzed 220 cases of this syndrome [6]. He concluded that its prevalence ranged from 20 to 60% of all infarctions depending on the particular population surveyed with electrocardiograms or by autopsy.

I. ELECTROCARDIOGRAPHIC STUDIES

One of the problems in assessing the frequency of silent infarctions is in their definition. Unlike transient episodes of silent myocardial ischemia that can be documented during exercise tests, radionuclide proeedures, etc., the unrecognized infarctions are not witnessed at the time they occur — though this may change with the widespread use of 24-hour ambulatory electrocardiographic monitoring. Reliance on patients' memory of possible cardiac symptoms is not the best type of data, nor are physicians' office notes sufficient. In the final analysis, we are left with electrocardiographic evidence of a myocardial infarction that occurred at some point between two ECG examinations. Nevertheless, several groups have attempted to assess the frequency of this phenomenon from the tracings. Probably the best example of these surveys is the Framingham Study, a long-term prospective study of cardiovascular disease which began in 1948 in Framingham, Massachusetts, under the auspices of the National Institutes of Health. In this study, a standard cardiovascular examination was performed twice a year on 5209 subjects who ranged from 30 to 62 years at time of entry into the study. Cardiovascular endpoints were noted on these examinations, as well as by reviewing admission data to the town's hospital. The initial report on unrecognized infarctions was published in 1970 [7] and supplemented in 1973 [8] and 1984 [9]. The last report represents a 26-year follow-up. At this time, over 26% of infarctions in men and 34% in women were unrecognized (Table 1). Of these half were truly silent, while in the other half some atypical symptoms were present but were not sufficient for either the patient or physician to consider that an infarction was occurring. What this report also shows is that these unrecognized infarctions were uncommon in patients with prior angina.

Other groups have also studied silent infarctions with the electrocardiogram. Another large study, that of the Western Collaborative Group, found a 30% rate of unrecognized infarction [10]. Studies are not confined to the United States. Medalie and Goldbourt [11]

Table 1 Proportion of Myocardial Infarctions Unrecognized (by Age and Sex). Framingham Study, 26-Year Follow-Up

Age (years)	MIs Unrecognized (%)	
	Men	Women
35-44	16.6	0
45-54	17.8	35.3
55-64	26.4	40.0
65-74	37.8	32.4
75+	30.0	30.2
Total	26.3	34.5

(From W. B. Kannel and R. D. Abbott. In *Silent Myocardial Ischemia* [W. Rutishauser and H. Roskamm, eds.], Springer-Verlag, Berlin, 1984, pp. 131-137.)

performed a prospective analysis in 9509 healthy government employees in Israel. Almost 40% of the subsequent 427 infarctions in this group were unrecognized. One difference between this study and that of the Framingham group was that these ECGs were read independently of prior tracings. This might tend to overestimate the number of unrecognized infarctions. Like the Framingham study, half of the unrecognized infarctions were totally silent. Also, like the Framingham study, age and hypertension [12] were significantly associated with the development of unrecognized infarctions (Figure 1).

II. AUTOPSY STUDIES

In addition to the reports cited earlier [2-5], more pertinent pathological studies have recently been made available comparing the extent of coronary narrowing and size of the healed infarct in these patients. Cabin and Roberts [13] studied 61 patients with a healed transmural myocardial infarction. Medical records were reviewed in detail and the patients were divided into two groups according to the presence (33 patients) or absence (28 patients) of a clinical history of acute myocardial infarction. Patients with equivocal or

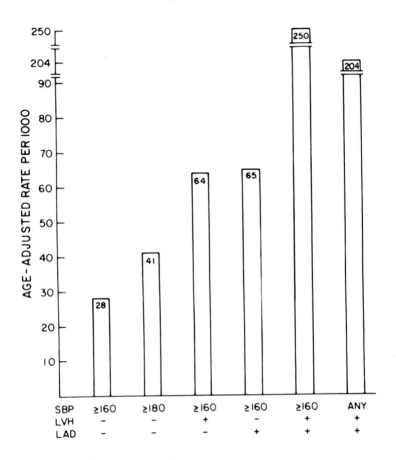

Figure 1   Five-year incidence of unrecognized (silent) myocardial infarction related to systolic blood pressure (SBP), left ventricular hypertrophy (LVH) and left axis deviation (LAD). (From J. H. Medalie and U. Goldbourt. *Ann. Intern. Med.*, *84*:256, 1976.)

Table 2 Clinical Findings in 33 Patients with Clinically Recognized and in 28 with Clinically Unrecognized Acute Myocardial Infarction (MI) and Healed Transmural Infarction at Necropsy

	Clinically Recognized Acute MI (33 Patients)		Clinically Unrecognized Acute MI (28 Patients)		p value
	n	%	n	%	
Age (yr)					
Mean	61	—	60	—	NS
Range	27–81	—	25–82	—	NS
Male–female ratio	25:8	—	21:7	—	NS
Angina pectoris	14	42	6	21	NS
Chronic congestive heart failure	14	42	9	32	NS
Systemic hypertension	11	33	12	43	NS
Diabetes mellitus (adult onset)	5	15	12	43	<0.05
Mode of death					
Sudden	13	39	6	21	NS
Acute MI	8	24	7	25	NS
Chronic congestive heart failure	5	15	1	4	NS
Cardiac operation	2[a]	6	2[b]	7	NS
Cardiac catheterization	2	6	1	4	NS
Noncardiac	3	9	11	39	<0.01

[a]Coronary artery bypass grafting in 1 and left ventricular aneurysmectomy in 1.
[b]Coronary artery bypass grafting in both.
(From H. S. Cabin and W. C. Roberts. Am. J. Cardiol., 50:677, 1982.)

Table 3   Myocardial Infarct (MI) Size and Location in 33 Patients with and in 28 without a Clinical History of Acute MI and a Healed Transmural MI at Necropsy

Clinical History of Acute MI	Patients (n)	MI Size (%)		Number of Patients with Major (Minor)[a] Involvement of Each Left Ventricular Wall by MI			
		Range	Mean	Anterior	Posterior	Septal	Lateral
+	33	1-55	17	16 (1)	15 (3)	1 (12)	1 (14)
0	28	1-23	7	5 (1)	22 (1)	1 (8)	0 (9)
p value	—		< 0.001	< 0.01	< 0.025	NS	NS

[a]For each patient, major involvement refers to the left ventricular wall with the most scarring and minor involvement refers to 1 or more additional walls with scarring. In all but 3 patients the anterior or posterior wall of left ventricle was the site of major involvement.
(From H. S. Cabin and W. C. Roberts. Am. J. Cardiol., 50:677, 1982.)

Table 4   Number of Major Epicardial Coronary Arteries (CA) Narrowed 76 to 100% in Cross-Sectional Area (XSA) by Atherosclerotic Plaque in 33 Patients with and 28 without a History of Acute Myocardial Infarction (MI) and a Healed Transmural MI at Necropsy

Clinical History Acute MI	Patients (n)	Total CA (n)	Patients with CA Narrowed 76-100% in XSA										Mean CA per Patient Narrowed 76-100%
			LM		LAD		LC		R		Totals		
+	33	132	6	18	32	97	23	70	32	97	93	70	2.8
0	28	112	8	29	24	86	21	75	28	100	81	72	2.9
p value	—	—	NS		NS		NS		NS		NS		NS

LAD = left anterior descending; LC = left circumflex; LM = left main; R = right.
(From H. S. Cabin and W. C. Roberts. Am. J. Cardiol., 50:677, 1982.)

inadequate histories were excluded. The group with unrecognized infarcts had a significantly higher prevalence of death from non-cardiac causes, posterior wall infarcts and small infarctions, as well as diabetes (Tables 2 and 3). However, the extent of narrowing of the coronary arteries was similar, as was the involvement of the various vessels (Table 4). The authors also addressed the question of whether patients with unrecognized infarcts had angina less frequently than did patients with symptomatic infarctions. Their results suggested this was the case, but the differences were not statistically significant.

III. MECHANISMS TO EXPLAIN THE ABSENCE OF PAIN. IS DIABETES MELLITUS A FACTOR?

In Chapter 1, we discussed cardiac pain pathways, and in Chapter 2, possible alterations in pain sensibility during silent myocardial ischemia. In addition, some investigators have studied pain mechanisms in patients with silent infarctions. Procacci et al. [14] studied 18 such subjects. They tested their cutaneous pain thresholds in the arm and found them to be significantly higher than in normals, but not higher than in patients with painful infarctions. They also studied upper-limb ischemia via cuff inflation and again found different onsets of pain and altered pain patterns compared to normals. They chose the arm because of the similar peripheral innervation found in "referred" cardiac pain.

These authors did not evaluate the effect of diabetes mellitus but others have. For example, Bradley and Schonfeld [15] reported that 42 of 100 diabetic patients had painless infarctions compared with 6 of 100 nondiabetic patients. This relationship was confirmed in the previously cited autopsy study of Cabin and Roberts [13]. As seen in Table 2, there was a significantly increased prevalence of diabetes mellitus among the patients in the unrecognized infarct group (43%) compared with those in the recognized infarct group. However, in two epidemiologic studies cited earlier [9, 11], the association of diabetes with unrecognized myocardial infarction did not reach a statistical level.

Pathological involvement of the automic nervous system by diabetes was demonstrated by Faerman et al. [16]. Abnormal morphology was found in cardiac sympathetic and parasympathetic nerves (Figures 2–4). None of the changes were found in specimens

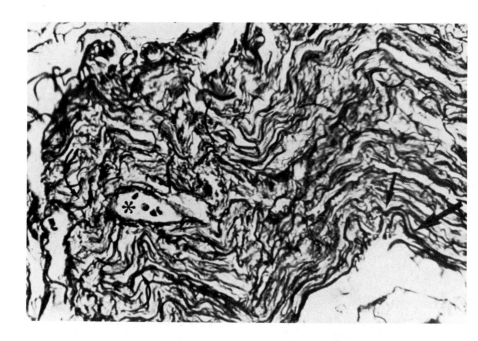

Figure 2   Abnormal appearance of a nerve fiber of a diabetic patient with painless myocardial infarction. Many fibers with hyperargentophilia, alterations of thickness and fragmentation (arrows).
Abnormally small number of fibers. A vasa nervorum with normal
wass (asterisk). Stain: trichrome and argentic impregnation.
×300. (From I. Faerman, E. Faccio, J. Milei, R. Nunez, M.
Jadzinsky, D. Fox, and M. Rapaport. *Diabetes*, *26*:1147, 1977.)

taken from a control group. These findings of a visceral neuropathy may help to explain the absence of pain during transient
ischemia, as well as during infarction. Raper et al. [17] postulated
that diabetes was responsible for painless infarction in one of four
cases that they reported as presenting to the hospital with acute
life-threatening cardiac illness. These patients came to the hospital because of complications of cardiac ischemia (such as pulmonary edema) but were pain-free. The other three patients did
not have diabetes but one had previous bypass surgery which may
have denervated part of the myocardium.

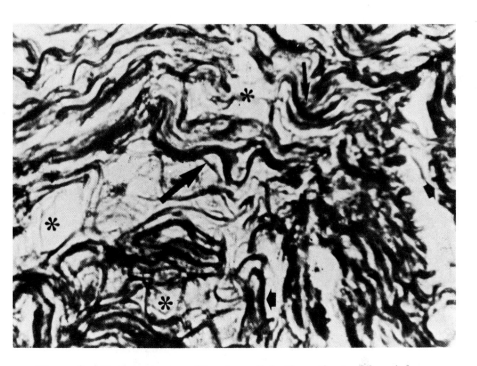

Figure 3   Abnormal nerve fiber in a diabetic patient with painless
myocardial infarction. Note the spindle shape of many of the
fibers (arrows), the interruption of fibers and the enlarged inter-
fibrillar spaces (asterisks). Trichrome and argentic impregnation .
× 1000. (From I. Faerman, E. Faccio, J. Milei, R. Nunez, M.
Jadzinsky, D. Fox, and M. Rapaport. *Diabetes, 26*:1147, 1977.)

Diabetes as a possible distinguishing feature of silent myocardial ischemia is discussed further in Chapter 7 of the next section
of this book.

IV. CONCLUSIONS

Thirty to forty percent of myocardial infarctions are silent or at
least clinically unrecognized. At autopsy the extent of coronary
artery disease is similar to that seen with symptomatic infarctions.
The etiology of painless infarctions is unclear, but the presence of
diabetes appears to be a factor in some studies.

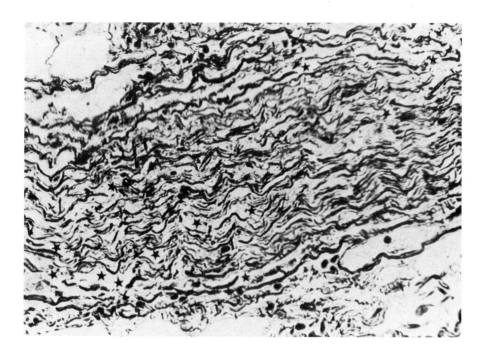

Figure 4   Diffuse abnormalities in a nerve fiber of the heart in a
diabetic patient with painless myocardial infarction. Note the
many fragmentations of the fibers (stars), hyperargentophilia and
smaller number of fibers. Trichrome and argentic impregnation.
×300. (From I. Faerman, E. Faccio, J. Milei, R. Nunez, M.
Jadzinsky, D. Fox, and M. Rapaport. *Diabetes, 26*:1147, 1977.)

REFERENCES

1. J. B. Herrick. Clinical features of sudden obstruction of the
    coronary arteries. *J.A.M.A., 59*:2015 (1912).
2. J. A. Kennedy. The incidence of myocardial infarction with-
    out pain in autopsied cases. *Am. Heart J., 14*:703 (1937).
3. L. D. Boyde and S. C. Weblow. Coronary thrombosis without
    pain. *Am. J. Med. Sci., 194*:814 (1937).
4. L. W. Gorham and S. J. Martin. Coronary artery occlusion
    with and without pain. *Arch. Intern. Med., 112*:812 (1938).

5. W. D. Stroud and J. A. Wagner. Silent or atypical coronary occlusion. *Ann. Intern. Med.*, *15*:25 (1941).

6. M. D. Roseman. Painless myocardial infarction: A review of the literature and analysis of 220 cases. *Ann. Intern. Med.*, *41*:1 (1954).

7. W. B. Kannel, P. M. McNamara, M. Feinleib, et al. The unrecognized myocardial infarction: 14 year follow-up experience in the Framingham study. *Geriatrics*, *25*:75 (1970).

8. J. R. Margolis, W. B. Kannel, M. Feinleib, et al. Clinical features of unrecognized myocardial infarction: 18 year follow-up: The Framingham study. *Am. J. Cardiol.*, *32*:1 (1973).

9. W. B. Kannel and R. D. Abbott. Incidence and prognosis of unrecognized myocardial infarction. Based on 26 years follow-up on the Framingham study. In *Silent Myocardial Ischemia* (W. Rutishauser and H. Roskamm, eds.), Springer-Verlag, Berlin, 1984, pp. 131–137.

10. R. H. Rosenman, M. Friedman, C. D. Jenkins, et al. Clinically unrecognized infarction in the Western Collaborative Study. *Am. J. Cardiol.*, *19*:776 (1967).

11. J. H. Medalie and U. Goldbourt. Unrecognized myocardial infarction: five-year incidence, mortality, and risk factors. *Ann. Intern. Med.*, *84*:526 (1976).

12. W. B. Kannel, A. L. Dannenberg, and R. D. Abbott. Unrecognized myocardial infarction and hypertension. The Framingham Study. *Am. Heart J.*, *109*:581 (1985).

13. H. S. Cabin and W. C. Roberts. Quantitative comparison of extent of coronary narrowing and size of healed myocardial infarct in 33 necropsy patients with clinically recognized and in 28 with clinically unrecognized ("silent") previous acute myocardial infarction. *Am. J. Cardiol.*, *50*:677 (1982).

14. P. Procacci, M. Zoppi, L. Padeletti, and M. Maresca. Myocardial infarction without pain. A study of the sensory function of the upper limbs. *Pain*, *2*:309 (1976).

15. R. F. Bradley and A. Schonfeld. Diminished pain in diabetic patients with myocardial infarction. *Geriatrics*, *17*:322 (1962).

16. I. Faerman, E. Faccio, J. Milei, R. Nunez, M. Jadzinsky, D. Fox, and M. Rapaport. Autonomic neuropathy and painless

myocardial infarction in diabetic patients: Histologic evidence of their relationship. *Diabetes, 26*:1147 (1977).

17. A. J. Raper, A. Hastillo, and W. J. Paulsen. The syndrome of sudden severe painless myocardial ischemia. *Am. Heart J., 107*:813 (1984).

III

DETECTION OF ASYMPTOMATIC CORONARY ARTERY DISEASE

7
What Can Be Learned from Standard Diagnostic Procedures?

Standard diagnostic procedures for evaluating suspected coronary artery disease in persons with chest pain include history taking, physical examination, blood lipid and glucose determinations, the resting ECG, and chest X rays and related procedures. Exercise testing — with or without associated radioisotopic procedures — is usually the next step after these standard procedures and is discussed in subsequent chapters. Obviously, screening asymptomatic populations for the presence of coronary artery disease is a more difficult undertaking and in this regard [1] not all of the above-mentioned procedures have the same value as they do in patients with chest pain syndromes.

I. HISTORY TAKING

This is of limited value since, by definition, the individual to be screened has no symptoms. (This, of course, does not include patients now asymptomatic but who have experienced a prior infarction.) At times, cardiologists will clearly recognize anginal "equivalents" that have been misdiagnosed by the patients (or their physicians) as gastrointestinal or neuromuscular complaints. Perhaps the most important information that truly asymptomatic individuals can provide, however, relates to their family history and/ or their own known coronary risk factors.

If a member of the individual's immediate family (i.e., parents, grandparents, aunts, uncles) died of cardiac (or unknown) causes or developed a myocardial infarction or angina before the age of 55, this should alert the cardiologist or internist to the possibility of latent coronary atherosclerosis. Since much of a "positive family history" is due to the prevalence of the three most important genetically determined risk factors (hypertension, diabetes mellitus, hypercholesteremia), patients should then be queried directly about the presence of these factors in their relatives — and themselves. Although cigarette smoking is not an inherited problem, smoking is another risk factor that can be part of a positive family history since patients who smoke encourage their children to do likewise merely by setting an example.

II. PHYSICAL EXAMINATION

Unless the patient has experienced a prior myocardial infarction with resulting left ventricular asynergy and its characteristic cardiac findings, the physical examination is usually negative. A fourth heart sound may be present even in individuals without prior infarctions, but this is too nonspecific a finding to be used by itself to diagnose coronary artery disease.

III. BLOOD TESTS

Abnormal blood glucose or lipid levels are recognized risk factors for the development of coronary artery disease. Whether they can be used as *indicators* of asymptomatic coronary artery disease is less clear.

Epidemiologic studies — such as that in Framingham, Massachusetts — have clearly shown the increased risk associated with increasing levels of serum cholesterol [2]. Other studies have examined the ratio of total cholesterol to high density lipoprotein (HDL) cholesterol. Williams et al. [3] studied 2568 asymptomatic men and found that a ratio of 4.0 or less identified a group with a very low prevalence of diseases, whereas a ratio of 8.0 or above identified a very high-risk group in relation to future cardiac events. Serum lipid levels have also been used to aid in the selection of subjects for coronary arteriography. Uhl et al. [4] found a ratio greater than 6.0 generated an odds ratio of 172/1 based on coronary angiographic results in 132 asymptomatic airmen with a positive exercise test. Only 2 of the 16 with coronary artery disease had a ratio less than 6.0, whereas only 4/102 persons with normal coronary angiographic findings had a ratio greater than 6.0. The ratio was a better discriminator than total cholesterol or HDL cholesterol levels (Figures 1 and 2). In a preliminary report, Kwiterovich et al. [5] investigated the elevated apoprotein levels of coronary artery disease in an asymptomatic population. Apoproteins are associated with cholesterol transport, and the major apoprotein B of low-density lipoproteins has previously been shown to be elevated in symptomatic individuals. In their report, Kwiterovich et al. studied plasma levels of various types of cholesterol and apoproteins in 68 asymptomatic siblings of 40 patients with premature coronary artery disease. Of the 19 siblings with a positive stress-thallium test, 10 had elevated apoprotein B levels. Bivariate analysis showed that apoprotein B was significantly more sensitive in this regard than other cholesterol and apoprotein measurements. As this study suggests, the presence of single or multiple risk factors combined with abnormal exercise responses

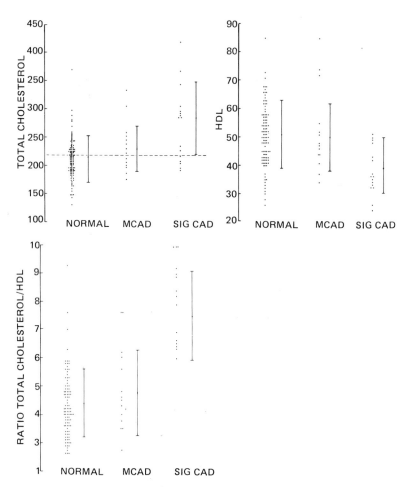

Figure 1   Values for total cholesterol, HDL cholesterol and choles-
terol/HDL cholesterol ratio in each of the patients plotted according
to angiographic classification (normal, minimal coronary artery
disease [MCAD] and significant coronary artery disease [SIG CAD]).
An arbitrary cutoff value for total cholesterol of 220 mg/100 ml is
represented by the dotted line. Total cholesterol and HDL cholesterol levels did not discriminate between those with significant
coronary artery disease and those with normal coronary angiograms. A cholesterol/HDL cholesterol ratio greater than 6.0 was
the best discriminator. (From G. S. Uhl, R. G. Troxler, J. R. Hickman, Jr., and D. Clark. *Am. J. Cardiol.*, *48*:903, 1981.)

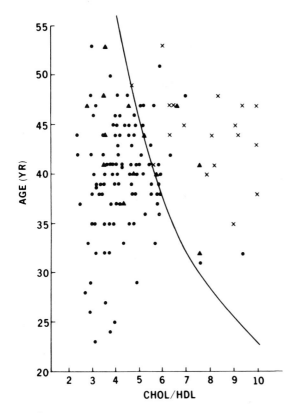

Figure 2 Graph plotting the cholesterol (CHOL)/HDL cholesterol
ratio versus age for each patient who underwent cardiac catheterization. The ratio and age appear to be independent risk factors.
The solid line plots the equation: age X (total cholesterol/HDL
cholesterol) = 230. It demonstrates that a simple equation can
separate normal subjects from patients with significant coronary
artery disease (CAD).   • = normal; ▲ = minimal CAD; x = significant CAD. (From G. S. Uhl, R. G. Troxler, J. R. Hickman, Jr.,
and D. Clark. *Am. J. Cardiol.*, *48*:903, 1981.)

Table 1   Angiographic Findings in 111 Aircrewmen with an
Abnormal Exercise Electrocardiogram Grouped According to
Annual Rest Electrocardiographic (ECG) Findings

Annual Rest ECG	n	Mean Age (%)	Significant Angiographic Coronary Disease (%)
Normal	34	44	23.5
Previous ST–T change but current ECG normal	21	43	23.8
Low amplitude T waves	24	42	25.0
ST segment abnormal	32	44	46.9

(From V. Froelicher, A. J. Thompson, R. Wolthius, et al. *Am. J. Cardiol.*, *23*:32, 1977.)

can also improve predictive value for coronary artery disease. This is discussed at greater length in Chapters 9 and 10.

IV.   THE RESTING ELECTROCARDIOGRAM

The standard baseline ECG obtained at rest is of value if it shows unequivocal evidence of new or old myocardial infarction. In totally asymptomatic individuals, one assumes the infarct was either silent, or painless enough not to warrant concern by the patient and/or his physician at the time. The finding of ST abnormalities alone suggests underlying coronary artery disease will be found in a relatively small number of subjects, but when combined with a positive exercise test, the predictive value increases to nearly 50%, which is higher than that observed with T wave changes alone (Table 1) [6]. Joy and Trump [7] concluded from their study of 103 asymptomatic men with minor ST segment abnormalities that the predictive value for coronary artery disease for these changes alone was about 8%, whereas it was 44% when combined with a positive exercise test. Changes with hyperventilation were not as impressive and these could not be used to separate presumably normal persons from those with coronary artery disease. This was also true of the U.S. Air Force studies [6]. In other Air

Force patients, the prevalence rate of coronary artery disease was 22% in asymptomatic airmen with new left bundle branch block and 18% in right bundle branch block [6].

Ventricular premature beats — either on resting ECGs or on Holter monitors — are not in themselves regarded as indicators, or predictors, of coronary artery disease if other evidence of organic heart disease is lacking [8].

Another approach to the ECG is computer analysis of the first and second integral of the voltage versus time (the "cardiointe-gram"). In a preliminary report [9] predictive accuracy was 74% in 186 patients who had also undergone cardiac catheterization and had normal resting ECGs. This device may be useful as a screening tool if results are confirmed in the future.

V. CHEST X RAYS AND RELATED PROCEDURES

The chest X ray is usually normal in this type of patient unless a prior infarction has occurred, or an ischemic cardiomyopathy has developed. Fluoroscopic screening for coronary artery disease (via detection of coronary artery calcification) is simple, rapid and in-expensive, but its reliability has been questioned, especially in older patients. In a preliminary study [10], Rifkin et al. studied 184 asymptomatic subjects with fluoroscopy and coronary angio-graphy. They found that coronary artery calcification was a strong marker for coronary artery stenosis in subjects under the age of 50 years but is a weak marker for those over the age of 60 years. Some groups have used the combination of fluoroscopy and stress testing as screening markers in asymptomatic populations. We will con-sider this in Chapter 10. Echocardiograms and radionuclide ven-triculography are also considered in Chapter 10 as adjuncts to the exercise test, since stress-related abnormalities of left ventricular wall motion are much more common than resting abnormalities in asymptomatic persons. One instrument that has been reported in a preliminary study to detect abnormal left ventricular function at rest is the cardiokymograph. The cardiokymograph is an electronic device that produces a representation of regional left ventricular wall motion. Zoltnick et al. [11] studied 287 asymptomatic sub-jects. They found an abnormal cardiokymograph to have a predic-tive value of 50%, equaling that of stress testing.

VI. CONCLUSIONS

Standard clinical procedures are of limited value as indicators of asymptomatic coronary artery disease, though coronary risk factors can help predict who will *subsequently* develop coronary artery disease.

REFERENCES

1. G. S. Uhl and V. Froelicher. Screening for asymptomatic coronary artery disease. *J. Am. Coll. Cardiol.*, *1*:946 (1983).
2. W. B. Kennell, W. P. Castelli, and T. Gordon. Cholesterol in the prediction of atherosclerotic disease: New perspective based on the Framingham Study. *Ann. Intern. Med.*, *90*:85 (1979).
3. P. Williams, D. Robinson, and A. Bailey. High density lipoprotein and coronary risk factors in normal men. *Lancet*, *1*: 72 (1979).
4. G. S. Uhl, R. G. Troxler, J. R. Hickman, Jr., and D. Clark. Angiographic correlation of coronary artery disease with high density lipoprotein cholesterol in asymptomatic men. *Am. J. Cardiol.*, *48*:903 (1981).
5. P. O. Kwiterovich, D. M. Becker, T. Pearson, D. J. Fintel, P. Bachorik, and A. Sniderman. HyperapoB is a potent predictor of occult coronary artery disease in asymptomatic relatives (abstr). *Circulation*, *70*(Suppl 11):313 (1984).
6. V. Froelicher, A. J. Thompson, R. Wolthuis, et al. Angiographic findings in asymptomatic aircrewmen with electrocardiographic abnormalities. *Am. J. Cardiol.*, *39*:32 (1977).
7. M. Joy and D. W. Trump. Significance of minor ST segment and T wave changes in the resting electrocardiogram of asymptomatic subjects. *Br. Heart J.*, *45*:48 (1981).
8. A. J. Moss. Clinical significance of ventricular arrhythmias in patients with and without coronary artery disease. *Prog. Cardiovasc. Dis.*, *23*:33 (1980).
9. L. E. Teichholz, M. Y. Steinmetz, D. Escher, M. V. Herman, D. V. Mahony, M. H. Ellestad, and S. Naimi. The cardiointegram: Detection of coronary artery disease in patients with normal resting electrocardiograms (abstr). *J. Am. Coll. Cardiol.*, *3*:598 (1984).

10. R. D. Rifkin, B. F. Uretsky, S. C. Sharma, E. D. Polland, D.
    A. Pietro, G. V. R. K. Sharma, P. S. Reddy, and A. F. Parisi.
    Fluroscopic screening for coronary artery disease (abstr).
    Circulation, *70*(Suppl 11):281 (1984).
11. J. M. Zoltick, J. Patton, J. Vogel, W. Daniels, J. L. Bedynek,
    and J. E. Davia. Cardiovascular screening evaluation to test
    for coronary artery disease in asymptomatic males over the
    age of 40 (abstr). *J. Am. Coll. Cardiol.*, *1*:638 (1982).

8

Ambulatory Electrocardiography (Holter Monitoring)

The 12-24-hour ambulatory electrocardiogram (popularly known as
the Holter monitor after its inventor) is widely used for the detection of arrhythmias, but it has gained increasing attention as a way
of detecting silent myocardial ischemia. The validity of this approach
has been questioned, however.

I. ARE ST SEGMENT CHANGES ON HOLTER MONITORS RELIABLE INDICATORS OF MYOCARDIAL ISCHEMIA?

The issue of whether or not ST segment changes recorded on Holter monitors are reliable indicators of myocardial ischemia has been a controversial one ever since continuous ambulatory monitoring was introduced in the 1960s. ST segments are labile and notoriously susceptible to hyperventilation, electrolyte abnormalities, drugs, etc. But there are also specific criticisms concerning the ambulatory ECG. Some of these involve technical considerations in recording of the electrocardiographic signal. The American Heart Association [1] has recommended a flat amplitude signal for frequency responses between 0.1 and 80 Hz, but many of the amplitude modulated (AM) ambulatory ECG monitoring systems amplify low-frequency information normally present in the ST segment. This can have the effect of overestimating the degree of ST segment depression relative to the height of the R wave. In addition to the concerns with frequency response curves, there is also the specific monitor to consider. Different systems will record standardized ST segment signals with different wave forms (Figure 1). Analysis of Holter tapes can also present difficulties. Recently developed computer programs for detecting transient ST changes appear to offer the best ways of analyzing the Holter tapes [2] (Figures 2 and 3).

With these caveats in mind, we can review some of the more important Holter studies. Stern and colleagues [3] first demonstrated ST segment abnormalities in a series of 80 patients with chest pain syndromes, normal resting electrocardiograms and normal exercise tests. Thirty-seven of the eighty patients had ischemic ST segment abnormalities (either elevation or depression) on their ambulatory recordings. Many of these episodes were unaccompanied by pain (Figure 4). In the initial 12-month follow-up period, 1 of these 37 patients developed a myocardial infarction; 23 others developed increasing chest pain or further ECG changes suggestive of coronary artery disease. Coronary arteriography was not performed in any of these patients. In another study, Stern and associates [4] studied 140 patients with chronic ischemic heart disease documented by anginal histories or myocardial infarctions. Ninety-seven of the one hundred forty patients had ST segment abnromalities during their daily activities. Some individuals (24%) had more ischemic episodes during sleep, while others

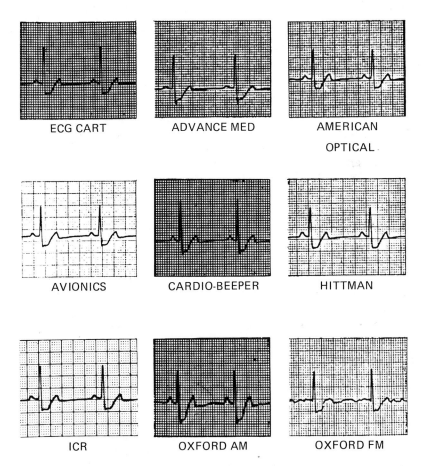

Figure 1 The representative output from one record/transmitter and one scanner/receiver of the input of the modified ECG simulator with 4-mm flat-line ST segment depression of 80 msec duration. Note the output from an HP 12-lead ECG cart (model 1541A) used as the standard. Note that the American Optical, Avionics and ICR systems gave good reproduction of the signal. Although the Hittman system reproduced the ST segment there was some attenuation of the terminal S wave. The Oxford AM gave considerably more than 4.0-mm ST segment depression. Advance Med and Cardio-Beeper had slightly upsloping ST segments. Note the baseline noise present on Oxford FM which limits clinical interpretation. (From D. A. Bragg-Remschel, C. M. Anderson, and R. A. Winkle. *Am. Heart J., 103*:20, 1982.)

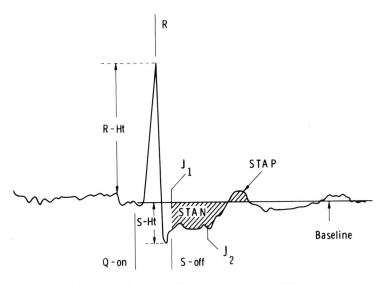

Figure 2   Diagram showing the variables identified and measured for each cardiac cycle by a computer system. J_1 = J point; J_2 = level of the ST segment 60 msec after the J point; R = R wave; R–Ht = R wave amplitude; S–Ht = S wave amplitude; Q-on = onset of Q wave; S-off = end of S wave; STAN = ST segment negative area; STAP = ST segment positive area. Heart rate is calculated from the RR interval. (From A. Gallino, S. Chierchia, G. Smith, M. Croom, M. Morgan, C. Marchesi, and A. Maseri. *J. Am. Coll. Cardiol.*, 4:245, 1984).

(38%) had a reduction in such episodes. In yet other studies [5], this group attempted to correlate the results of ambulatory monitoring with coronary arteriography: ambulatory ECGs identified nearly 80% of patients with angiographically documented coronary artery disease. The false-positive rate (positive ECG findings with normal coronary arteriograms) was only 13%.

Other groups have also attempted to correlate ambulatory ECGs with the results of coronary arteriograms. Crawford and colleagues [6] studied 70 patients (39 with and 31 without coronary artery disease) with 24-hour ambulatory monitors, exercise stress tests, as well as coronary arteriography. Twenty-four of the thirty-nine patients (62%) with coronary artery disease had ischemic

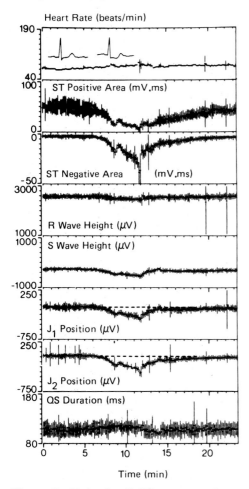

Figure 3   Episode of ST segment depression as represented by the computer printout. The values of each derived variable, calculated on a beat by beat basis, were averaged on 10-second periods and plotted against time with the corresponding values of the standard deviation. During ST depression, there is a decrease in ST segment positive area (due to a decrease in T wave amplitude), an increase in negative area (due to ST segment depression) and negative displacement of both J_1 and J_2. The two complexes at the top were retrieved from the computer digital tape and show the electrocardiographic pattern during the control period (left) and ischemia (right). (From A. Gallino, S. Chierchia, G. Smith, M. Croom, M. Morgan, C. Marchesi, and A. Maseri. *J. Am. Coll. Cardiol.*, *4*:245, 1984.)

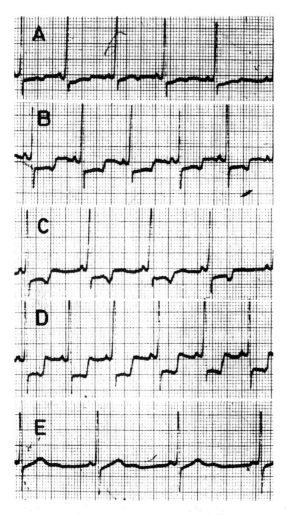

Figure 4   An example of the ST–T changes observed during 24-hour ambulatory ECG monitoring in a 56-year-old man. Slight ST–T abnormalities were noted during most of the day (panel A); increasing degrees of ST segment depression were observed after meals (panel B), at rest (panel C) and during walking (panel D). Only during sleep at night (panel E) was the ECG normal. Although the patient had apparent evidence of myocardial ischemia as shown in panels B, C, and D, he only experienced pain during walking (panel D). (From S. Stern and D. Tzivoni, *Am. Heart J.*, *91*:820, 1976.)

ST segment abnormalities on the 24-hour monitors. This compared to 26 patients (or 67%) who had positive stress tests. By contrast, in the 31 patients free of coronary artery disease, 19 (61%) had no ischemic abnormalities on 24-hour monitoring. The exercise stress test was negative in 23 of the 31 subjects (75%).

II. HOLTER MONITORING AND SILENT MYOCARDIAL ISCHEMIA

Most of the studies cited above dealt peripherally with the issue of silent myocardial ischemia. The first Holter study to specifically evaluate the significance of asymptomatic episodes was that of Schang and Pepine [7]. Twenty patients with angiographically confirmed coronary artery disease and positive exercise tests were each monitored for several 10-hour periods over the course of 16 months. In the total of 2826 hours of technically adequate recordings, 411 episodes of transient ST segment abnormalities were documented (Figure 5). Of the 411 episodes, 308 (or 75%) were asymptomatic. Most of these occurred during sleep, sitting or periods of slow walking (Figure 6) and at heart rates very much less than those at which patients complained of angina during their stress tests. Schang and Pepine indirectly "proved" that the silent ST segment episodes were truly ischemic by markedly reducing their frequency with prophylactic use of long-acting nitrate preparations. This was an important feature of their study, since, as noted previously, considerable criticism had been directed toward the use of the ST segment as a marker of ischemia.

The use of ambulatory monitoring for detecting silent ischemia via ST segment abnormalities in persons *not* known to have coronary artery disease has been questioned very strenuously. When Armstrong and Morris [8] evaluated 50 asymptomatic middle-aged men with treadmill exercise tests and ambulatory ECG monitoring and found evidence of "ischemic" ST segment changes in 15 of the 50 men (30%), they concluded that these were false-positive responses, similar to those observed in cases of mitral valve prolapse or neurocirculatory asthemia or in any condition where the autonomic nervous system can be overactive. Quyumi et al. [9] have also reported ST segment changes in presumably healthy men, but Deanfield et al. [10] found significant depression only rarely.

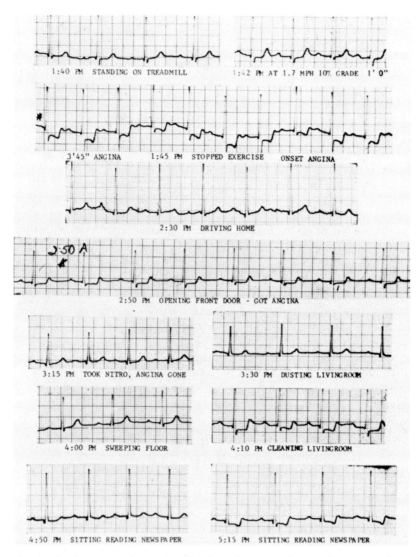

Figure 5 Another example of ST–T changes observed on ambulatory monitoring in a building manager. ECG changes occurred on an exercise test, during work, and at rest, but were not always accompanied by pain. (From S. J. Schang and C. J. Pepine. *Am. J. Cardiol.*, *39*:396, 1977.)

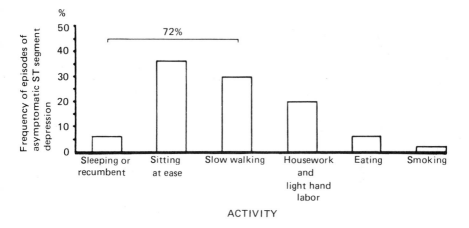

Figure 6   Activity at the onset of 310 asymptomatic episodes of ST depression. Almost three-fourths of these painless ischemic events occurred during very light activity. (From S. J. Schang and C. J. Pepine. *Am. J. Cardiol., 39*:396, 1977.)

Since, in patients with known coronary artery disease, there appears to be more acceptance of the ST segment as a marker of ischemia, it is reasonable to assume that an asymptomatic episode would carry the same weight as a symptomatic one. However, it was not until the study published by Deanfield and co-workers [11] appeared that this assumption gained acceptance. This study and its successor [12] succeeded in refuting much of the skepticism concerning the relative importance of symptomatic versus asymptomatic episodes in the same person. In 30 patients with stable angina and positive exercise tests, ambulatory ST segment monitoring was used to record episodes of transient ischemia during daily life. All patients had four consecutive days of monitoring, and in 20 patients long-term variability was evaluated by repeated 48-hour monitoring and exercise testing over an 18-month period. Of the 1934 episodes of horizontal or downsloping ST segment depression, only 470 (or 24%) were accompanied by angina — a figure almost identical to that of Schang and Pepine in their study published six years earlier. Physiologic validation of the ST segment change was an especially important part of their second

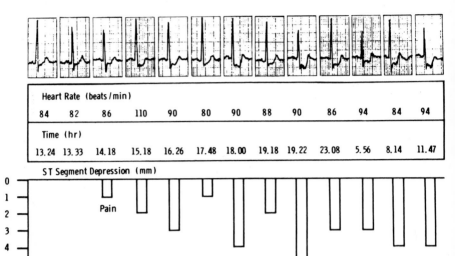

Figure 7　Typical 24 hour ambulatory electrocardiographic recording showing 11 episodes of ST depression, only one of which was accompanied by angina. The episodes occurred throughout day and night and lasted for up to 40 minutes. (From J. E. Deanfield, P. Ribiero, K. Oakley, S. Krikler, and A. P. Selwyn. *Am. J. Cardiol.* *54*:1195, 1984.)

study [12], which included 34 patients. That ischemia could occur without angina was documented by positron tomography (see Figure 13 in Chapter 4) with the occurrence of ST segment depression being consistently underestimated by symptoms. Heart rate increase was not common (Figure 7), suggesting transient increases in coronary vasomotor tone as a major contributor to myocardial ischemia — with or without symptoms — during daily life.

Another recent study has confirmed the frequency of silent ischemic episodes in patients with classic exertion-induced angina pectoris, as well as their occurrence at lower heart rates. This study, by Cecchi and colleagues [13], also found the number of silent episodes to outnumber the symptomatic ones. In their study of 39 patients with exertion-induced angina, they performed 24-hour Holter monitoring in addition to exercise testing. Coronary artery disease was confirmed by coronary arteriography in 31 pa-

Table 1   Ischemic Episodes During Holter Monitoring (39 patients)

Patients (no.)	Total	Episodes (no.)	
		Symptomatic	Asymptomatic
7	0	—	—
8	25	25	—
15	105	29	76
9	40	—	40
Total	170	54	116

(From A. C. Cecci, E. V. Dovellini, F. Marchi, P. Pucci, C. M. Santoro, and P. F. Fazzini. *J. Am. Coll. Cardiol.*, *1*:934, 1983.)

tients, and 16 patients had a prior myocardial infarction. Of the 39 patients, 32 had ST depression during ambulatory monitoring (Table 1). Fifteen of the thirty-two patients had both symptomatic and asymptomatic episodes (with asymptomatic episodes being three times as frequent); in this study the duration and degree of ST segment depression was greater during the asymptomatic episodes (Table 2). Deanfield et al. [11] noted the duration of the asymptomatic episodes to be shorter than the symptomatic ones (Figure 8), though there was considerable overlap in values and the myocardial perfusion defects appeared similar. Cecchi et al. [13] also reported that patients who took longer to register chest pain during treadmill stress testing had a greater ratio of symptomatic to painless episodes of myocardial ischemia on 24-hour monitoring (Table 3). Their studies suggested that the severity of the ischemic episode, i.e., the amount of myocardium at jeopardy is an important factor in determining whether a specific ischemic episode would be symptomatic or not (see also Chapter 4). By contrast, Kunkes et al. [14] reported that patients with multivessel disease (and presumably *more* myocardium at jeopardy) had a higher frequency of silent ischemic episodes than did patients with one-vessel disease (Figure 9).

III. CONCLUSIONS

The use of Holter monitoring to document silent myocardial ischemia in patients experiencing both symptomatic and asympto-

Table 2   24 Hour Holter Monitoring: Duration of Ischemic Attacks and Magnitude of Maximal ST Depression

	Patients (no.)	Episodes (no.)	Type of Episodes	Duration of Episodes	Mean Magnitude of Maximal ST Depression
All patients	32	54	Symptomatic	7' ± 5'42"	3.3 ± 1.7 mm
		116	Asymptomatic	4'12" ± 2'30"	2.5 ± 1 mm
		Total 170		(p < 0.001)	(p < 0.001)
Patients who experienced only symptomatic or asymptomatic episodes	8	25	Symptomatic	5'12" ± 3'50"	2.3 ± 0.9 mm
	9	40	Asymptomatic	4'33" ± 3'	2.7 ± 1.2 mm
		Total 65		(p > 0.05)	(p > 0.05)
Patients who exhibited both symptomatic and asymptomatic episodes	15	29	Symptomatic	8'36" ± 6'35"	4.3 ± 1.7 mm
		76	Asymptomatic	4'06" ± 2'15"	2.4 ± 1.0 mm
		Total 105		(p < 0.001)	(p < 0.001)

(From A. C. Cecci, E. V. Dovellini, F. Marchi, P. Pucci, C. M. Santoro, and P. F. Fazzini. *J. Am. Coll. Cardiol.*, *1*:934, 1983.)

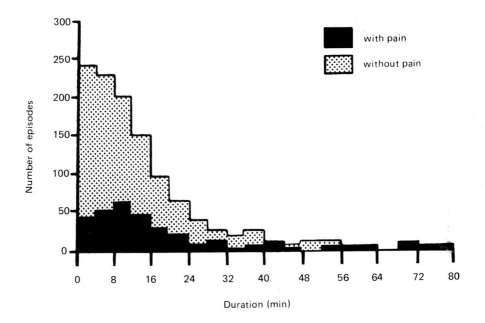

Figure 8 Histogram showing duration of symptomatic and asymptomatic episodes of ST depression. (From J. E. Deanfield, A. P. Selwyn, S. Chierchia, A. Maseri, P. Ribiero, S. Krikler, and M. Morgan. *Lancet*, 2:753, 1983.)

Table 3 Results of Stress Testing and Holter Monitoring

Stress Testing		Holter Monitoring		
Patients (no.)	Finding	Patients (no.)	Episodes (no.)	Ratio Between Symptomatic and Asymptomatic Episodes
			Symptomatic Asymptomatic	
11	Angina precedes or coincides with ST depression	11	27 17	1:0.62
10	ST depression precedes angina by 10 to 60 seconds	8	11 12	1:1.09
18	ST depression precedes angina by more than 60 seconds	13	16 87	1:5.43

(From A. C. Cecci, E. V. Dovellini, F. Marchi, P. Pucci, C. M. Santoro, and P. F. Fazzini. *J. Am. Coll. Cardiol., 1*:934, 1983.)

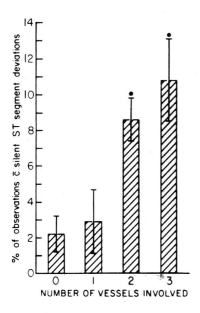

Figure 9 Correlation of silent ST segment deviations with the extent of coronary artery disease. Hatched bars represent the percentage of observation with silent ST segment deviations on the ambulatory ECG for each grade of coronary artery disease. Note how this percentage increases with the extent of coronary artery disease. * = significantly different from 0-1-vessel disease ($p < 0.001$). (From S. H. Kunkes, A. D. Pichard, H. Smith, Jr., R. Gorlin, M. V. Herman, and J. Kupersmith, *Am. Heart J.*, *100*: 813, 1980.)

matic episodes seems well established. Still uncertain, however, is whether ST changes seen in otherwise healthy individuals have the same connotation. Consequently, the role of routine Holter monitoring in detecting coronary artery disease in the asymptomatic population is unclear.

REFERENCES

1. H. V. Pipberg, R. C. Arzbaecher, A. S. Berson, S. A. Briller, D. A. Brody, N. C. Flowers, D. B. Geselowitz, E. Lepeschkin,

C. G. Oliver, O. H. Schmitt, and M. Spach. Recommendations for standardization of leads and of specifications for instruments in electrocardiography and vectorcardiography: Report of the Committee on Electrocardiography, American Heart Association. *Circulation*, *52*:11 (1975).

2. A. Gallino, S. Chierchia, G. Smith, M. Croom, M. Morgan, C. Marchesi, and A. Maseri. Computer system for analysis of ST segment changes on 24 hour Holter monitor tapes: Comparison with other available systems. *J. Am. Coll. Cardiol.*, *4*:245 (1984).

3. S. Stern and D. Tzivoni. Early detection of silent ischaemic heart disease by 24-hour ECG monitoring during normal daily activity. *Br. Heart J.*, *36*:481 (1974).

4. S. Stern and D. Tzivoni. Dynamic changes in the ST-T segment during sleep in ischemic heart disease. *Am. J. Cardiol.*, *32*:17 (1973).

5. S. Stern, D. Tzivoni, and Z. Stern. Diagnostic accuracy of ambulatory ECG monitoring in ischemic heart disease. *Circulation*, *52*:1045 (1975).

6. M. H. Crawford, C. A. Mendoza, R. A. O'Rourke, D. H. White, C. A. Boucher, and J. Gorwit. Limitations of continuous ambulatory electrocardiogram monitoring for detecting coronary artery disease. *Ann. Intern. Med.*, *89*:1 (1978).

7. S. J. Schang and C. J. Pepine. Transient asymptomatic S–T segment depression during daily activity. *Am. J. Cardiol.*, *39*: 396 (1977).

8. W. F. Armstrong and S. N. Morris. The ST segment during ambulatory electrocardiographic monitoring. *Ann. Intern. Med.*, *98*:249 (1983).

9. A. A. Quyumi, C. Wright, and K. Fox. Ambulatory electrocardiographic ST segment changes in healthy volunteers. *Br. Heart J.*, *50*:460 (1983).

10. J. E. Deanfield, P. Ribiero, K. Oakley, S. Krikler, and A. P. Selwyn. Analysis of ST segment changes in normal subjects: Implications for ambulatory monitoring in angina pectoris. *Am. J. Cardiol.*, *54*:1321 (1984).

11. J. E. Deanfield, A. P. Selwyn, S. Chierchia, A. Maseri, P. Ribiero, S. Krikler, and M. Morgan. Myocardial ischemia during daily life in patients with stable angina: Its relation to symptoms and heart rate changes. *Lancet*, *2*:753 (1983). (1983).

12. J. E. Deanfield, M. Shea, P. Ribiero, C. M. deLandsheere, R.
     A. Wilson, P. Horlock, and A. P. Selwyn. Transient ST seg-
     ment depression as a marker of myocardial ischemia during
     daily life. *Am. J. Cardiol.*, *54*:1195 (1984).
13. A. C. Cecci, E. V. Dovellini, F. Marchi, P. Pucci, C. M. Santoro,
     and P. F. Fazzini. Silent myocardial ischemia during ambula-
     tory electrocardiographic monitoring in patients with effort
     angina. *J. Am. Coll. Cardiol.*, *1*:934 (1983).
14. S. H. Kunkes, A. D. Pichard, H. Smith, Jr., R. Gorlin, M. V.
     Herman, and J. Kupersmith. Silent ST segment deviations
     and extent of coronary artery disease. *Am. Heart J.*, *100*:
     813 (1980).

9
Exercise Testing

The exercise test is an established procedure for assessing ischemic responses, arrhythmias and cardiac performance in persons with known or suspected heart disease. In addition, many epidemiologic studies have been performed to evaluate the accuracy of exercise electrocardiographic testing in predicting the occurrence of overt cardiac events in asymptomatic populations. It is only recently (within the last five years) that the exercise test has been used as a procedure to screen asymptomatic individuals in order to identify those persons who warrant further non-invasive or invasive testing because of an abnormal exercise response. This latter approach considers the exercise electrocardiogram as an *indicator* of myocardial ischemia, rather than as a risk factor for the development of coronary artery disease.

I. EXERCISE TESTS AS PREDICTORS OF FUTURE CARDIAC EVENTS

One of the earliest and largest of the epidemiologic studies was that initiated in 1971 by Bruce and colleagues [1, 2] in Seattle. In this prospective community study of symptom-limited maximal exercise testing, more than 4000 persons clinically free of heart disease were registered between 1971 and 1974. Annual follow-up surveillance of subsequent primary coronary artery disease (defined as admission to a hospital for evaluation or treatment) was continued until the beginning of 1981. Thus, this study provides a unique 10-year experience for evaluating the interactive value of exercise test predictors combined with the usual coronary risk factors (hypertension, hyperlipidemia, diabetes, cigarette smoking) and a family history of premature coronary artery disease in the 3611 men and 547 women enrolled in this study. Mean age of the men was 45.5 ± 8.4 (SD) years; for the women it was 49.1 ± 9.0 years. The standard Bruce protocol for symptom-limited maximal exercise using progressive increments in speed and gradient on a motor-driven treadmill was employed. The most common cause for stopping the tests was fatigue. Patients were divided into subgroups based on presence of conventional risk factors and four abnormal exercise predictors. These included (1) chest pain during the test; (2) inability to complete stage 2 of the protocol; (3) maximal heart rate less than 90% of age-predicted normal vlaue (based on the formulae $y = 227 - 1.067$ [age in years for men] and $y = 206 - 0.597$ [age in years for women]); and (4) development of 1 mm or more of horizontal or downsloping ST depression for at least 1 minute into the recovery period. Event rates for cardiac events per 1000 person-years of follow-up were calculated. Prior to applying the results of exercise testing, the annual incidence rate of total cardiac events was 0.35% in asymptomatic healthy

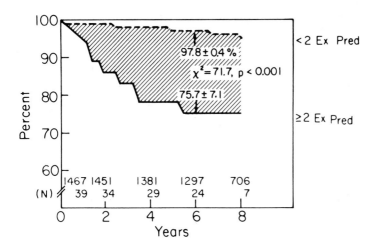

Figure 1 Stepwise assessment of survival without any primary coronary heart disease events in three groups of middle-aged men and
women initially free of coronary heart disease manifestations.
Shaded areas represent differences in survival rates attributable to
the detection of less than two or more than two exercise predictors.
(From R. A. Bruce, K. F. Hossack, T. A. DeRouen, and V. Hofer.
J. Am. Coll. Cardiol., 2:565, 1983.)

men and 0.31% in women. When the interaction of any conventional risk factor and two or more of the exercise predictors was
considered, the annual risk of cardiac death (for men and women
combined) increased from 0.12% to 9.61% (p < 0.05). Six-year
survival rates decreased from 97.8 ± 0.4% to 75.7 ± 7.1 (p < 0.001)
in this subgroup when a life-table analysis was performed (Figure 1).
    Other studies have used ST segment depression alone as a pre-
dictor of future cardiac events. For example, Ellestad and Wan [3]
collected follow-up data on 2700 patients, including 323 who had
previous infarcts. They found that by using a 1.5-mm criterion
for ST segment depression, they could demonstrate a significant
difference between positive and negative responders in terms of
future cardiac events such as death, myocardial infarction or progressive angina (9.5%/year vs. 1.7%/year). The adverse prognosis
seen with a positive stress test was especially marked in those individuals who had experienced a prior myocardial infarction (Figure

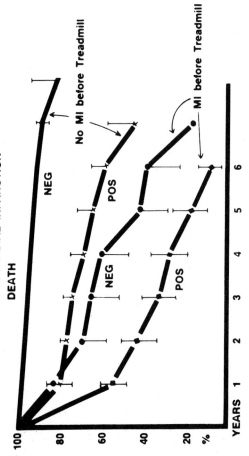

COMBINED EVENTS:
PROGRESSION OF ANGINA
MYOCARDIAL INFARCTION
DEATH

NEG-No MI Before Tread	Sample#	1127	836	718	611	461	369	265	153	23
	Year	0	1	2	3	4	5	6	7	8
POS-No MI Before Tread	Sample#	427	303	214	168	133	97	49	20	2
	Year	0	1	2	3	4	5	6	7	8
NEG TREAD MI Before Tread	Sample#	92	70	56	43	33	24	13	4	
	Year	0	1	2	3	4	5	6	7	
POS TREAD MI Before Tread	Sample#	231	139	88	62	38	24	9	5	
	Year	0	1	2	3	4	5	6	7	

Figure 2 The incidence of all coronary events in the negative and positive ST responders who had not had a previous infarction is compared with the negative and positive responders who had a previous myocardial infarction. (From M. H. Ellestad and M. K. C. Wan. *Circulation, 51*:363, 1975, with permission from the American Heart Association.)

Table 1 Correlation of Combining All Three Positive Criteria (ST,
R-wave and Exercise Duration) vs. Absence of Criteria with
Development of Coronary Heart Disease Within 5 Years in Men
Older Than 40 Years

	ST Positive and Increase or No Change in R Wave and Duration ⩽ 5 Minutes	ST Negative and Decrease in R Wave and Duration > 5 Minutes
CHD	5[a] (100%)	12 (5.8%)
No CHD	0 (0%)	194 (94.2%)

Sensitivity 29.4%; specificity 100%; predictive value of a positive test 100%;
risk ratio 17.2.
[a]$p < 0.001$.
CHD = coronary heart disease
(From W. H. Allen, S. W. Aronow, P. Goodman, and P. Stinson. *Circulation*,
62:522, 1980.)

2). Allen et al. [4] studied 888 clinically normal men and women.
They did not evaluate conventional risk factors but did assess multiple exercise predictors, including ST segment depression, abnormal
R-wave response and exercise duration of 5 minutes or less. All
three factors were present in five men aged 40 or over; all subsequently developed cardiac events (Table 1). Similarly, absence of
all three factors provided 94% predictive accuracy for absence of
cardiac events in the 206 men who were aged 40 or over. These
predictive values were not reliable, however, in men under 40 or in
women.

The most recent study of this type was performed by Giagnoni
et al. [5]. These investigators controlled their study for the effect
of conventional risk factors so that they could isolate the ST segment response as a predictor of ischemic events. Between 1971 and
1974, they identified 10,723 subjects (8866 men and 1857 women)
who were apparently free of heart disease and hypertension; 135
persons had bicycle ergometer exercise-induced ST depression of 1
minute or more on two exercise electrocardiograms. For each person, two or three controls with negative exercise tests and matched

Table 2   Occurrence of Coronary Events in 135 Cases and 379
Controls

	Cases	Controls	Total
	no. (%)	no. (%)	no. (%)
Coronary events			
Present	21 (15.55)	13 (3.43)	34 (6.61)
Absent	114 (84.45)	336 (96.57)	480 (93.39)
Total	135 (100)	379 (100)	514 (100)
Relative risk	4.53		

(From E. Giagnoni, M. B. Secchi, S. C. Wu, A. Morabito, L. Oltrona, S.
Mancarella, N. Volpin. L. Fossa, L. Bettazzi, G. Arangio, A. Sachero, and G.
Folli. *N. Engl. J. Med.*, *309*:1085, 1983.)

for age, sex, occupation and conventional risk factors were selected.
Follow-up for cardiac events (angina, myocardial infarction, sudden death) was conducted for a period of six years (Table 2). The
incidence of coronary events was very low in the controls (0.8% for
the first five years) as compared to 10.37% in the study group
(Figure 3). This difference was higher than that observed in the
second five years. Although, as expected, the conventional risk
factors were also prognostic indicators in this study, the authors
concluded that the positive exercise electrocardiogram was an
independent risk predictor. In a subsequent letter to the editor
of the *New England Journal of Medicine* [6], these results were
criticized on a cost-benefit basis since it required exercise testing
in over 10,000 healthy individuals to produce 135 persons (1.2%)
with a positive test, of whom only 21 or (19%) had coronary
events over a five-year period. In their reply, Giagnoni et al. drew
attention to the fact that they were not advocating mass screening
but rather suggested confining exercise testing to males over 45
with "high levels" of conventional risk factors. This is also my
approach.

Exercise-induced ventricular premature beats, as opposed to
ST segment depression or duration of exercise, do not appear to
be reliable predictors of cardiac events in asymptomatic persons
[7].

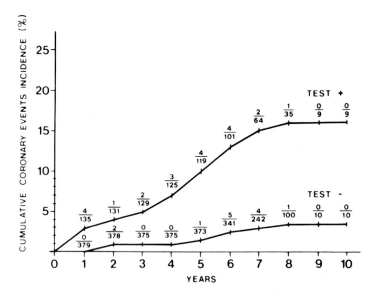

Figure 3   Cumulative curves for the incidence of coronary events in cases (TEST +) and in controls (TEST —). For each year of follow-up the number of coronary events observed (numerator) and the number of subjects exposed to the risk (denominator) are indicated. Relative risk as determined by Cox's regression model is 5.55 (95% confidence limits, 2.75 to 11.22); as determined by logistic matched-set analysis, 5.03 (95% confidence limits, 2.41 to 10.49). (From E. Giagnoni, M. B. Secchi, S. C. Wu, A. Morabito, L. Oltrona, S. Mancarella, N. Volpin, L. Fossa, L. Bettazzi, G. Arangio, A. Scachero, and G. Folli. *N. Engl. J. Med., 309*:1085, 1983.)

II.   EXERCISE TESTS AS INDICATORS OF ASYMPTOMATIC CORONARY ARTERY DISEASE

In my opinion, what is overlooked in the epidemiologic studies cited is that the abnormal ST segment response may be more than merely a risk factor that *predicts* disease. An abnormal response may instead be an *indicator* that latent disease is already present. To confirm this hypothesis, it would be necessary to submit positive responders to coronary arteriography, i.e., "case finding."

However, the frequency of false-positive responses in an asymptomatic population is high, based on low disease prevalence, i.e., Bayes' theorem [8], discussed at length in Chapter 10. For example, Eriksson et al. [9], in their studies of Norwegian factory workers, selected 115 men out of a cohort of 2014 presumably healthy men based on a positive exercise test. Of the 115, 105 underwent coronary angiography but only 69 had significant disease (75% stenosis). In Froelicher's study of U.S. Air Force personnel [10], 1390 men were exercised and 135 had abnormal tests. Only 35 (25.4%) had significant coronary artery disease. When Hopkirk et al. [11] added more study subjects to Froelicher's original group and then investigated the predictive value of exercise duration plus persistence of ST depression plus the depth of ST depression, they achieved almost 90% predictive accuracy for coronary artery disease, and a predictive value only slightly less than that for multivessel disease (84%). The three test variables (i.e., those with the highest "likelihood ratio") were 3 mm or more of ST segment depression, persistence of ST depression 5 minutes after exercise, and total duration of exercise of less than 10 minutes. The combination of any two of these three exercise risk predictors plus one of the conventional risk factors yielded the predictive value noted earlier (Table 3).

Other investigators [12–14] have also examined the degree of ST depression and its persistence into the recovery period with or without hypotension. They agree that the greater the ischemic change, the more likely asymptomatic or minimally symptomatic patients will have severe disease. For example, in the study by Hamby et al. [14] (Table 4), 27 patients had positive exercise tests. Of the six with an abnormal blood pressure response, five (or 83%) had left main or triple-vessel disease. By contrast, only 9 of the 21 persons (43%) with a normal blood pressure response had this finding on angiography.

Changes in the R wave on the electrocardiogram have also been looked at specifically in studies of U.S. Air Force personnel; 65 men with coronary artery disease and 190 normal subjects formed the study population [15] (Table 5). R-wave amplitude changes were evaluated in bipolar leads X, Y and Z. Exercise-induced changes in R-wave height (diminution or no change) increased the specificity of detecting coronary artery disease in asymptomatic men over ST segment criteria alone, but the sensitivity was poor and the overall predictive value not enhanced. These results differ

Table 3 Combination of Exercise Test Variables and Conventional Risk Factors for the Detection of Any Coronary Disease and Multivessel Disease

Combination	Any Coronary Disease (n = 65)		Multivessel Disease (50 R; n = 33) (70 R; n = 28)			
	Sensitivity (%)	Predictive Value (%)	Sensitivity (%)		Predictive Value (%)	
			50 R	70 R	50 R	70 R
1	6	67	30	36	71	71
2	28	52	45	50	68	64
3	17	92	33	39	85	85
4	37	89	55	64	84	81

Combination 1 = 0.3 mV horizontal or downsloping ST depression beginning by stage II and exercise time less than 10 minutes; combination 2 = 0.3 mV horizontal or downsloping ST depression beginning by stage II and 0.1 mV ST depression persisting 6 minutes after exercise; combination 3 = combination of 1 and 2; combination 4 = presence of one or more conventional risk factors and at least two of the exercise risks mentioned above; 50R, 70R = 50%, 70% luminal reduction.
(From J. A. C. Hopkirk, G. S. Uhl, J. R. Hickman, Jr., J. Fischer, and A. Medina. *J. Am. Coll. Cardiol.,* 3:887, 1984.)

Table 4 Relation of Exercise Blood Pressure Response to Main Left or Triple-Vessel Coronary Disease, or Both

	Patient Group			
	A (n = 27)	B (n = 36)	C (n = 57)	Total (n = 120)
Abnormal blood pressure response	6	9	21	36[a]
Left main or triple vessel coronary disease (%)	5 (83%)	8 (89%[a])	17 (81%)	30 (83%)
Normal blood pressure response	21	27	36	84[a]
Main left or triple vessel coronary disease, or both (%)	9 (43%)	8 (30%[a])	25 (69%)	42 (50%)

[a] $p < 0.01$ (comparison of percent of patients in group B with left main or triple vessel coronary disease, or both, in the subgroups with abnormal and normal blood pressure responses). Group A = no angina; Group B = mild angina; Group C = moderate angina. (From R. I. Hamby, E. T. Davison, J. Hilsenrath, S. Shanies, M. Young, D. H. Murphy, and I. Hoffman. J. Am. Coll. Cardiol., 3:1375, 1984.)

Table 5 Diagnostic Accuracy of Different Criteria in Detecting Different Angiographic Definitions of Coronary Artery Disease (50 or 70% Reduction [R] in Luminal Diameter or Multivessel Disease [MVD])[a]

	Sensitivity (%)			Specificity (%)			Predictive Value (%)		
	50 R	70 R	MVD	50 R	70 R	MVD	50 R	70 R	MVD
ST depression	—	—	—	—	—	—	25	18	14
R wave amplitude at stress									
↑ X	28	28	31	87	86	86	42	30	28
↑ Y	32	33	32	81	80	81	37	26	32
↑ ΣXY	22	24	26	88	88	88	38	30	34
↓ Z	82	97	95	20	5	16	26	2	16

[a]Multivessel disease = coronary disease, defined as 50% reduction of luminal diameter, in two or three major vessels.
↑ = increase; ↓ = decrease. X, Y and Z refer to X, Y and Z bipolar leads.
(From J. A. C. Hopkirk, G. S. Uhl, J. R. Hickman, Jr., and J. Fischer. *J. Am. Coll. Cardiol.*, 3:821, 1984.)

from those of Yiannikas et al. [16], who have found that the R wave response was more helpful than ST segment responses. As noted earlier, Allen et al. [4] also used the R wave response in combination with other ECG measurements to improve diagnostic accuracy in asymptomatic men.

III. CONCLUSIONS

Abnormal exercise test responses in asymptomatic populations appear to be reliable *predictors* of future cardiac events, but it is only recently that their value as *indicators* of occult coronary artery disease has been evaluated with coronary arteriographic studies. Because of the problem of false-positive responses in an asymptomatic population, stress tests should be considered as screening procedures for coronary artery disease only in those individuals with one or more risk factors and/or family histories of premature coronary artery disease. The abnormal test is likely to be a "true-positive" response when other abnormalities besides ST changes are present.

REFERENCES

1. R. A. Bruce, T. A. DeRouen, and K. F. Hossack. Value of maximal exercise tests in risk assessment of primary coronary heart disease events in healthy men: Five years' experience of the Seattle Heart Watch Study. *Am. J. Cardiol.*, *46*:371 (1980).
2. R. A. Bruce, K. F. Hossack, T. A. DeRouen, and V. Hofer. Enhanced risk assessment for primary coronary heart disease events by maximal exercise testing: 10 years' experience of Seattle Heart Watch. *J. Am. Coll. Cardiol.*, *2*:565 (1983).
3. M. H. Ellestad and M. K. C. Wan. Predictive implications of stress testing: Follow-up of 2700 subjects after maximum treadmill stress testing. *Circulation*, *51*:363 (1975).
4. W. H. Allen, S. W. Aronow, P. Goodman, and P. Stinson. Five-year follow-up of maximal treadmill stress test in asymptomatic men and women. *Circulation*, *62*:522 (1980).
5. E. Giagnoni, M. B. Secchi, S. C. Wu, A. Morabito, L. Oltrona, S. Mancarella, N. Volpin, L. Fossa, L. Bettazzi, G. Arangio, A. Sachero, and G. Folli. Prognostic value of exercise EKG

testing in asymptomatic normotensive subjects: A prospective matched study. *N. Engl. J. Med.*, *309*:1085 (1983).

6. D. Nicklin and D. J. Balaban. Exercise EKG in asymptomatic normotensive subjects. *N. Engl. J. Med.*, *310*:853 (1984).

7. C. K. Nair, W. S. Aronow, M. H. Sketch, T. Pagano, J. D. Lynch, A. N. Moose, D. Esterbrooks, V. Runco, and K. Ryschon. Diagnostic and prognostic significance of exercise-induced premature ventricular complexes in men and women: A four year follow-up. *J. Am. Coll. Cardiol.*, *1*:1201 (1983).

8. R. Detrano, J. Yiannikas, E. E. Salcedo, G. Rincon, R. T. Go, G. Williams, and J. Leatherman. Bayesian probability analysis: A prospective demonstration of its clinical utility in diagnosing coronary disease. *Circulation*, *69:*541 (1984).

9. J. Erikssen, I. Enge, R. Forfang, and D. Storstein. False positive diagnostic tests of coronary angiographic findings in 105 presumably healthy males. *Circulation*, *54*:371 (1976).

10. V. F. Froelicher, A. J. Thompson, M. R. Longo, Jr., J. H. Triebwasser, and M. C. Lancaster. Value of exercise testing for screening asymptomatic men for latent coronary artery disease. *Prog. Cardiovasc. Dis.*, *18*:265 (1976).

11. J. A. C. Hopkirk, G. S. Uhl, J. R. Hickman, Jr., J. Fischer, and A. Medina. Discriminant value of clinical and exercise variables in detecting significant coronary artery disease in asymptomatic men. *J. Am. Coll. Cardiol.*, *3*:887 (1984).

12. D. S. Blumental, J. L. Weiss, E. D. Mellits, and G. Gerstenblith. The predictive value of a strongly positive stress test in patients with minimal symptoms. *Am. J. Med.*, *70*:1005 (1981).

13. E. C. Lozner and J. Morganroth. New criteria to enhance the predictability of coronary artery disease by exercise testing in asymptomatic subjects. *Circulation*, *56*:799 (1977).

14. R. I. Hamby, E. T. Davison, J. Hilsenrath, S. Shanies, M. Young, D. H. Murphy, and I. Hoffman. Functional and anatomic correlates of markedly abnormal stress tests. *J. Am. Coll. Cardiol.*, *3*:1375 (1984).

15. J. A. C. Hopkirk, G. S. Uhl, J. R. Hickman, Jr., and J. Fischer. Limitation of exercise-induced R wave amplitude changes in detecting coronary artery disease in asymptomatic men. *J. Am. Coll. Cardiol.*, *3*:821 (1984).

16. J. Yiannikas, J. Marcomichelakis, P. Taggart, B. H. Keely, and
     R. Emanuel. Analysis of exercise-induced changes in R wave
     amplitude in asymptomatic men with electrocardiographic
     ST–T changes at rest. *Am. J. Cardiol.*, *47*:238 (1981).

10
Combining the Exercise Test with Other Procedures

We combine the exercise test with other procedures in order to increase the reliability of detecting asymptomatic coronary artery disease. This is necessary because of the frequency of false-positive test responses, which is a function of Bayes' theorem. This theorem was alluded to in the preceeding chapter but several points deserve further emphasis.

I. BAYES' THEOREM

Bayes' theorem states that test results cannot be adequately inter-
preted without knowing the prevalence of the disease in the population under study. This is called the pretest likelihood (or prior
probability) of disease, as opposed to the posttest likelihood (or
posterior probability). Definitions and equations for these terms
are as follows:

Pretest likelihood (*prior probability*) is defined as the probability
of disease in a subject to be tested

$$= \frac{\text{number of patients with disease in the test population}}{\text{total number of patients in the test population}} \quad (1)$$

Posttest likelihood (*posterior probability*) is defined as the
probability of disease in a subject showing a given test result

$$= \frac{\text{number of patients with disease showing a given test result}}{\text{total number of subjects showing the test result}} \quad (2)$$

Bayes' theorem helps to explain the well-known observation that
a small proportion of normal persons will have a "false-positive"
response; i.e., they will have an abnormal test response but will
prove to be normal on more exact study. A good example is an
abnormal exercise test response that is suggestive of coronary
artery disease in a person who subsequently undergoes coronary
angiography and is found to have normal coronary arteries. In
short, the predictive value of any less-than-perfect test, such as the
exercise stress test, is reduced to an extent that is related in part
to the fraction of normal persons in the study population [1].

Epstein [2] gives two examples to illustrate this point. Key
terms are sensitivity, specificity and predictive value. These are
defined as follows with appropriate equations also provided:

Sensitivity is defined as the probability a patient with disease
will have a given test result

$$= \frac{\text{number of patients with disease with a given test result}}{\text{total number of diseased subjects tested}} \quad (3)$$

Specificity is defined as the probability a patient without disease
will not have the given test result

$$= \frac{\text{number of disease-free subjects not showing the test result}}{\text{total number of disease-free subjects tested}} \quad (4)$$

Predictive value of a positive test is defined as the probability
that a patient has disease, given a positive test outcome

$$= \frac{\text{number of patients with disease}}{\text{total number of patients with a positive test}} \qquad (5)$$

Predictive value of a negative test is defined as the probability
that a patient does not have disease, given a negative test outcome

$$= \frac{\text{number of subjects without disease}}{\text{total number of subjects with a negative test}} \qquad (6)$$

Assuming exercise tests have a sensitivity of 75% and a specificity
of 85%, what are the chances that a positive test in an *asymptomatic*
person (with a 3% pretest likelihood of coronary artery disease)
truly indicates coronary artery disease? The answer is that the
positive test's predictive value (or posttest likelihood) of disease
being present is 14%. By contrast, the same positive test result
in a person *with angina* (and thus a 90% pretest likelihood of
coronary artery disease) yields a 98% posttest likelihood. The
predictive value of a negative test is inverse to that of a positive
test. The complete spectrum of pre- and posttest likelihoods of
the exercise test predicting coronary artery disease is depicted
in Figure 1. The posttest likelihoods are highest in those individuals with a high pretest likelihood and vice versa. The low predictive value in asymptomatic subjects has led investigators to
search for other ways of increasing the posttest likelihood. One
way is to construct a "family" of ST segment depression curves
as in Figure 2. We now no longer look upon the exercise test as
merely providing a "yes or no" statement regarding the presence
of coronary artery disease, but as providing a continuum of risk
based on different probability estimates. A "very positive" test,
i.e., one with more than 2.5 mm of ST depression, greatly increases
the posttest likelihood of coronary artery disease.

II. ADDING OTHER PROCEDURES INCREASES POSTTEST LIKELIHOOD

When *conventional risk factors* are taken into consideration, a high-
risk subgroup can be identified in which a positive exercise test has
more validity than in a low-risk group. Several groups have used
data from the *Coronary Risk Handbook* based on the Framingham

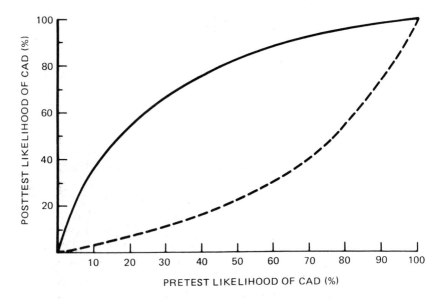

Figure 1 Influence of pretest likelihood of coronary artery disease (CAD) on the posttest likelihood of coronary artery disease. ——— = positive test (sensitivity 75%); – – – = negative test (specificity 85%). (From S. E. Epstein, *Am. J. Cardiol.*, *46*:491, 1980.)

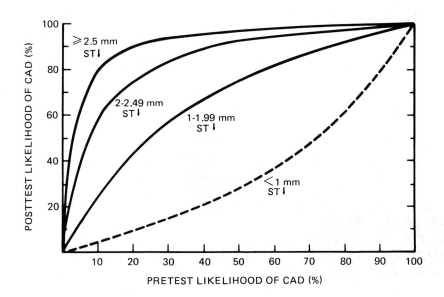

Figure 2   Family of ST segment depression curves (based on data derived from Diamond and Forrester [3]) and likelihood of coronary artery disease (CAD). ST↓ segment depression. (From S. E. Epstein. *Am. J. Cardiol.*, *46*:491, 1980.)

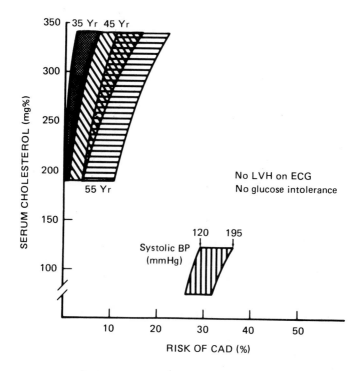

Figure 3   Effect of age, serum cholesterol and blood pressure (BP) on risk of coronary artery disease (CAD) in nonsmoking men 35 to 55 years of age. (The graph is based on data derived from the Framingham Study, in which the cholesterol values were obtained using the Abell-Kendall method. Most direct and automated cholesterol determinations give values 5–15% above that given in this graph.) ECG = electrocardiogram; LVH = left ventricular hypertrophy. (From S. E. Epstein. *Am. J. Cardiol.*, *46*:491, 1980.)

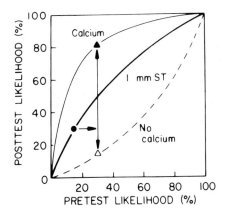

Figure 4   Influence of serial tests on posttest likelihood. The closed circle represents a patient with a pretest likelihood of 15 per cent (*x* axis) and a 1.0-mm depression of the ST segment after a stress test (heavy solid line). The resultant posttest likelihood is 27% (*y* axis). If cardiac fluoroscopy showed calcification of one coronary vessel (light solid line), the resultant posttest likelihood would rise (↑) to 79% (▲). If no calcification was observed (dashed line), the likelihood would fall (↓) to 14% (△). Note that the posttest likelihood from the first test becomes the pretest likelihood of the second test (horizontal arrow). (From G. A. Diamond and J. S. Forrester. *N. Engl. J. Med.*, *300*:1350, 1979.)

Study to provide relevant data. As seen in Figure 3, a 55-year-old man with a cholesterol level of 350 mg% and a systolic blood pressure of 195 mmHg would have a 20% pretest risk of coronary artery disease. With a positive exercise test, posttest likelihood could increase to 50–90% depending on the degree of ST segment depression.

When a second independent test is employed, the posttest likelihood from the exercise test becomes the pretest likelihood for the second test. An example is the demonstration of *coronary artery calcification* by fluroscopy, as depicted by Diamond and Forrester [3] in Figure 4. This particular observation is based partly on the work of Langou et al. [4], who have shown that the presence of coronary artery calcification is a powerful predictor

Table 1   Predictive Accuracy of Coronary Artery Calcification at
Fluoroscopy and Abnormal Exercise Stress Test

	No. Pts.	Significant CAD	CAD
Coronary calcification + abnormal exercise test	13	12	13
Predictive accuracy		92%	100%

(From R. A. Langou, E. K. Huang, M. J. Kelley, and L. S. Cohen. *Circulation*, *62*:1196, 1980.)

of coronary artery disease in asymptomatic men with a positive
exercise test. Langou et al. [4] screened 120 middle-aged males
free of clinical heart disease. Of the original group, 108 completed
the submaximal exercise protocol by achieving at least 90% of
their age-predicted maximal heart rate; these subjects made up the
study population. Sixteen subjects had a positive exercise test; 13
(81%) also had at least one calcified artery on fluoroscopy. By contrast, only 13 (35%) of the 37 subjects with coronary artery calcification had a positive exercise test. Cardiac catheterization was
performed in the 13 men with both a positive exercise test and
coronary calcification. As depicted in Table 1, one subject had
<50% luminal stenosis; all the rest had at least 75% luminal steno-
sis in one vessel with five persons having two-vessel disease and
three having three-vessel disease. Thus, the predictive accuracy
obtained by combining both noninvasive tests was 92%.

The influence of other serial tests besides cardiac fluoroscopy
on posttest likelihood has also been studied. Diamond et al. [5]
evaluated other noninvasive tests including the stress cardiokymograph, which is used for the detection of precordial regional left
ventricular dysfunction (noted previously in Chapter 7), and stress
thallium-201 scintigraphy for assessment of exercise-induced
regional myocardial hypoperfusion. The greater the number of
abnormal responses observed in a given patient, the greater the
predictive accuracy for coronary artery disease and especially
multivessel disease. Of the 974 patients studies in this manner,

278 (29%) were asymptomatic. A computer assisted program (called CADENZA) was used to analyze and report the results of the various tests (Table 2).

Epstein [2] also considered serial testing with *radionuclide procedures* since they have a higher predictive value than the exercise ECG alone. He reasoned that the combination of a positive exercise ECG and either an abnormal thallium perfusion scan or radionuclide ventriculogram would markedly increase the predictive value of the exercise test, although he cautioned that sensitivity and specificity of these tests in asymptomatic persons might well be different from that in symptomatic patients. Figure 5 is an example of this combined approach. The attractiveness of these radionuclide procedures is based on several studies of asymptomatic persons. Caralis et al. [6] found that 22 persons out of 3496 developed 2 mm or more ST segment depression on exercise testing. Of the 22 persons, 15 agreed to undergo thallium-201 exercise scintigrams: 10 were abnormal. Nolewajka et al. [7] found less promising results in their study of 58 asymptomatic men studied. Of the five men with abnormal thallium scans, subsequent coronary arteriography in three was normal. Uhl et al. [8] studied 191 airmen with abnormal exercise ECGs. Predictive value of the ECG was 21%, compared to 75% for scintigraphy. They felt the thallium test was a good second-line screening procedure. In a subsequent study [8] they compared the thallium-201 myocardial scintigram to the radionuclide ventriculogram. Again, all testing was done at the U.S. Air Force School of Aerospace Medicine; 32 airmen with abnormal exercise ECGs had both thallium scintigrams and radionuclide ventriculograms. Thirteen patients had angiographically documented coronary artery disease; 12 had abnormal thallium scans; 11 had reduced ejection fractions at maximal exercise. Table 3 compares the sensitivity and specificity of the two procedures.

On the basis of these observations, serial testing procedures have been advocated for use in U.S. Air Force personnel, as described by Uhl and Froelicher [9]. After initial history, physical examination and resting ECG are performed, a fasting biochemical profile is obtained, and a risk factor index calculated based on Framingham data. Men with positive exercise tests then would undergo cardiac fluoroscopy and thallium perfusion scintigraphy before being considered for cardiac catheterization. These authors

Table 2 Variables Analyzed by CADENZA

Variable	Measurement Interval	Conditional Variable
History		
Age (yr)	Continuous	—
Sex	Male. female	—
Chest discomfort	AS. NA. AA. TA	Age. sex
Systolic BP (mm Hg)	Continuous	Sex
Cholesterol (mg/dl)	Continuous	Age. sex
Currently smoking	Yes. no	Sex
Glucose intolerance	Yes. no	Sex
Rest ECG	Normal. abnormal	Sex
ECG stress test		
Duration of exercise (min)	Continuous	—
Magnitude of ST depression (mm)	< 0.5. 0.5. 1.0. 1.5. 2.0. > 2.5	Sex. rest ECG
Slope of ST segment	Upsloping. horizontal. downsloping	Rest ECG
R wave amplitude change (mm)	Continuous	—

Fluoroscopy		
No. of calcified vessels	0, 1, 2, 3	Age
Cardiokymography		
Rest pattern	I, II, III.	—
Postexercise pattern	I, II, III	Rest pattern
Thallium scintigraphy		
Type of defect	None, fixed, reversible	—
Magnitude of defect	Mild, moderate, severe	Type of defect
Pulmonary uptake	None, mild/moderate, moderate/severe	—
Technetium scintigraphy		
Rest ejection fraction (%)	Continuous	—
Peak exercise ejection fraction (%)	Continuous	—

AA = atypical angina; AS = asymptomatic; BP = blood pressure; ECG = electrocardiogram; I = inward systolic motion; II = mid-systolic outward motion; III = holosystolic outward motion; NA = nonanginal discomfort; TA = typical angina. (From G. A. Diamond, H. M. Staniloff, J. S. Forrester, B. H. Pollack, and H. J. C. Swan. *J. Am. Coll. Cardiol. 1*:444, 1983.)

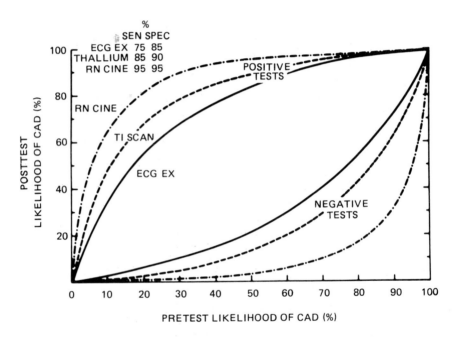

Figure 5 Probability of coronary artery disease (CAD). Comparison of electrocardiographic exercise testing (ECG EX), thallium perfusion scanning (TI SCAN) and radionuclide cineangiography (RN CINE). (Sensitivity [SEN] and specificity [SPEC] values are approximations derived from published series.) (From S. E. Epstein. *Am. J. Cardiol., 46*:491, 1980.)

Table 3 Comparison of Thallium Scintigraphy and Radionuclide Angiography

	Thallium 201		Ejection Fraction		Wall Motion		Ejection Fraction + Wall Motion
	Normal	Abnormal	Normal	Abnormal	Normal	Abnormal	Abnormal
Normal	18	1	16	3	18	1	1
Coronary artery disease	1	12	2	11	5	8	7
Sensitivity	92%		85%		62%		
Specificity	95%		85%		95%		

(From G. G. Uhl, T. N. Kay, and J. R. Hickman, Jr. *J. Cardiac. Rehabil.*, 2:118, 1982.)

Table 4   Criteria for Primary Cardiovascular Screen Failure in the
U.S. Army Over-Forty Program[a]

Framingham risk index of 5% or greater

Abnormal cardiovascular history or examination

Electrocardiogram abnormality
  (LVH, interventricular conduction defects, ST–T–wave changes,
  etc.)

Fasting blood sugar $\geq$ 115 mg/dl

[a]Any one abnormality requires secondary screening. LVH = left ventricular
hypertrophy.
(From J. M. Zoltick, H. A. McAllister, and J. L. Bedynek, Jr. *J. Cardiac
Rehabil.*, 4:530, 1984.)

have stressed the importance of lipid screening, citing the U.S. Air
Force studies described in Chapter 7, in which the ratio of total
cholesterol to high-density lipoprotein (HDL) cholesterol was a
useful predictor of disease. Only 42 (9.5%) of 440 men with a
normal exercise test had a ratio greater than 6.0; by contrast, 87%
of those with coronary artery disease had this finding for an odds
ratio of 172 to 1 [10]. The U.S. Army also has a similar cardiovascular screening program (11) (Table 4).

At the Johns Hopkins Hospital, serial testing procedures are
used to identify high risk subgroups in families with early coronary artery disease. Hypertension and hyperlipidemia in asymptomatic siblings was strongly correlated with positive stress thallium
tests. In one subgroup, for example, men over the age of 40 with
a systolic blood pressure greater than 150 mmHg had an 82% prevalence of positive stress thallium tests [12]. In this preliminary
report, coronary arteriographic findings were not presented.

III. CONCLUSIONS

Noninvasive detection of asymptomatic coronary artery disease is
best approached with a variety of procedures that can confirm an
abnormal stress test, since the next step — cardiac catheterization —
should only be performed when there is a very high suspicion that
latent coronary atherosclerosis is present.

REFERENCES

1. R. D. Rifkin and W. B. Hood, Jr. Bayesian analysis of electrocardiographic exercise stress testing. *N. Engl. J. Med.*, *297:* 681 (1977).
2. S. E. Epstein. Implications of probability analysis on the strategy used for noninvasive detection of coronary artery disease: Role of single or combined use of exercise electrocardiographic testing, radionuclide cineangiography and myocardial perfusion imaging. *Am. J. Cardiol.*, *46*:491 (1980).
3. G. A. Diamond and J. S. Forrester. Analysis of probability as an aid in the clinical diagnosis of coronary artery disease. *N. Engl. J. Med.*, *300*:1350 (1979).
4. R. A. Langou, E. K. Huang, M. J. Keeley, and L. S. Cohen. Predictive accuracy of coronary artery calcification and abnormal exercise test for coronary artery disease in asymptomatic men. *Circulation*, *62*:1196 (1980).
5. G. A. Diamond, H. M. Staniloff, J. S. Forrester, B. H. Pollack, and H. J. C. Swan. Computer-assisted diagnosis in the non-invasive evaluation of patients with suspected coronary artery disease. *J. Am. Coll. Cardiol.*, *1*:444 (1983).
6. D. G. Caralis, I. Bailey, H. L. Kennedy, and B. Pitt. Thallium-201 myocardial imaging in evaluation of asymptomatic individuals with ischaemic ST segment depression on exercise electrocardiogram. *Br. Heart J.*, *42*:452 (1979).
7. A. J. Nolewaijka, W. J. Kostuk, J. Howard, et al. Thallium stress myocardial imaging: An evaluation of fifty-eight asymptomatic males. *Clin. Cardiol.*, *4*:135 (1981).
8. G. S. Uhl, T. N. Kay, and J. R. Hickman, Jr. Comparison of exercise radionuclide angiography and thallium perfusion imaging in detecting coronary artery disease in asymptomatic men. *J. Cardiac. Rehabil.*, *2*:118 (1982).
9. G. S. Uhl and V. Froelicher. Screening for asymptomatic coronary artery disease. *J. Am. Coll. Cardiol.*, *1*:946 (1983).
10. G. S. Uhl, R. G. Troxler, J. R. Hickman, Jr., and D. Clark. Relation between high density lipoprotein cholesterol and coronary artery disease in asymptomatic men. *Am. J. Cardiol.*, *48*:903 (1981).
11. J. M. Zoltick, H. A. McAllister, and J. L. Bedynek, Jr. The United States Army Cardiovascular Screening Program. *J. Cardiac Rehabil.*, *4*:530 (1984).

12. D. M. Becker, T. Pearson, D. J. Fintel, D. M. Levine, and L. C. Becker. Risk factors identify high risk subgroups in families with early coronary heart disease (CHD). (abstr). *Circulation,* *70*(Suppl II):127 (1984).

11
Cardiac Catheterization

Cardiac catheterization that includes coronary arteriography (and usually left ventriculography) is still the accepted standard for the diagnosis of coronary artery disease. The number of cardiac catheterizations performed in the United States in 1980 was estimated to exceed 200,000, although indications for performing the procedure are still unsettled [1]. Because of this uncertainty, there is considerable controversy when a patient with asymptomatic coronary artery disease is detected via the noninvasive procedures discussed in Chapters 7 through 10, and coronary arteriography is considered to confirm the diagnosis. This controversy is most marked in totally asymptomatic persons and less so in those who are asymptomatic following a myocardial infarction. In those individuals with episodes of both symptomatic and asymptomatic myocardial ischemia, there is the least amount of controversy.

I. INDICATIONS FOR CARDIAC CATHETERIZATION IN TOTALLY ASYMPTOMATIC PERSONS

Ambrose [1] concluded that coronary arteriography "appears warranted in patients with objective evidence of significant ischemia at low work loads even though they are asymptomatic or minimally symptomatic. The purpose of catheterization is to identify those patients with significant coronary artery disease, so that appropriate therapy can be instituted if considered necessary." Before proceeding to catheterization, Ambrose emphasizes the need for a confirmatory radionuclide procedure in addition to a positive exercise test. This is in keeping with Conti's philosophy [2], among others, and it is certainly one that I concur with. The flow diagram that Conti uses to illustrate the subsequent evaluation of asymptomatic patients with a positive exercise test is depicted in Figure 1. In summary, these authors and myself feel that a positive exercise test should be followed by another independent demonstration of myocardial ischemia (abnormal thallium-201 scintigram or radionuclide ventriculogram) or demonstration of coronary artery calcification on fluoroscopy before proceeding to cardiac catheterization, an invasive procedure with small but definite associated morbidity and mortality.

Of course, not all physicians agree with this approach. Some "question the justification for the wide case-finding effort of subjecting asymptomatic persons to coronary arteriography . . . unless

Who needs coronary angiography?

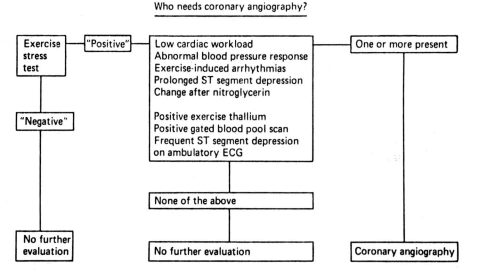

Figure 1   Flow diagram to illustrate one approach to evaluation of asymptomatic patients with a positive stress test. (From C. R. Conti. *Adv. Cardiol.*, *27*:181, 1980.)

unusual findings suggest an especially poor prognosis" [3]. Others take a middle of the road position that appears to leave open the possibility of coronary arteriographic study in appropriate patients with abnormal noninvasive tests [4, 5].

II.   INDICATIONS FOR CARDIAC CATHETERIZATION AFTER A MYOCARDIAL INFARCTION

Epstein et al. [6] have proposed a schema to identify patients who should undergo cardiac catheterization after a myocardial infarction (Figure 2). In addition to patients who are symptomatic with angina or congestive heart failure, they also recommend coronary arteriography in uncomplicated patients with adequate left ventricular function and inducible ischemia, i.e., ST segment depression and/or a fall in radionuclide ejection fraction. This recommendation is based on the adverse short-term prognosis associated with these findings. Veenbrink et al. [7] also used the exercise test response as a guide in their asymptomatic patients.

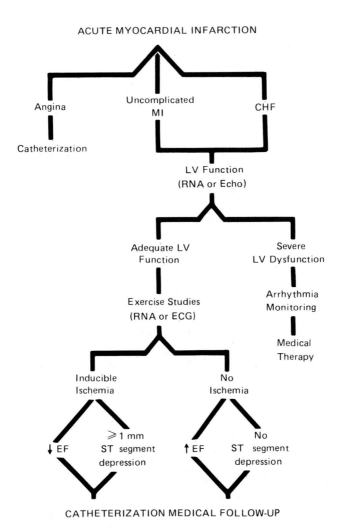

ACUTE MYOCARDIAL INFARCTION

Angina

Catheterization

Uncomplicated
MI

CHF

LV Function
(RNA or Echo)

Adequate LV
Function

Severe
LV Dysfunction

Exercise Studies
(RNA or ECG)

Arrhythmia
Monitoring

Medical
Therapy

Inducible
Ischemia

No
Ischemia

↓ EF   ≥ 1 mm
ST segment
depression

↑ EF   No
ST segment
depression

CATHETERIZATION MEDICAL FOLLOW-UP

Figure 2 Strategy for identifying patients who should undergo
cardiac catheterization after acute myocardial infarction. The
strategy is based on clinical assessment, evaluation of left ventricular
(LV) function by radionuclide angiography (RNA) or echocardiography, arrhythmia analysis, and stress testing. MI denotes acute
myocardial infarction, CHF overt congestive heart failure and EF
ejection fraction. (From S. E. Epstein, S. T. Palmeri, and R. E.
Patterson. *N. Engl. J. Med.*, *307*:1487, 1982.)

Table 1 Coronary Arteriographic Findings

Left main disease	0
Left main equivalent	2 (6%)
Left anterior descending stenosis	22 (71%)
Inferior MI[a]	11
Anterior MI	11
Three vessel disease	9 (29%)
Two vessel disease	10 (32%)
Single vessel disease	10 (32%)
Normal	2 (6%)
Coronary artery aneurysms	1
Anomalous circumflex from right coronary artery	1
Absent collateral vessels	10 (32%)

[a]One proximal and nine distal to the first septal perforator.
(From R. K. Mautner and J. H. Phillips. *Cardiovasc. Diag.*, 7:1, 1981.)

Mautner and Phillips [8] have a similar approach. They studied 31 patients, nine (29%) of whom were found to have triple-vessel disease (Table 1). Chaitman [9] found triple-vessel disease in 8 of 37 patients (22%), while Miller et al. [10] found this degree of obstruction in 38 of 84 patients (45%). Turner et al. [11] studied 117 patients with angiography — 61 of whom were asymptomatic, i.e., uncomplicated — and found triple-vessel disease in 14 (29%), but also found left main disease in four (7%) (Table 2). Despite this high frequency of severe disease (36%), Turner et al. did *not* recommend routine coronary arteriography after a myocardial infarction because of the "uncertainty of bypass surgery in prolonging life" in this subgroup of patients. In an accompanying editorial, Rahimtoola [12] enthusiastically endorsed this conservative approach.

III. INDICATIONS FOR CARDIAC CATHETERIZATION IN PATIENTS WITH BOTH SYMPTOMATIC AND ASYMPTOMATIC EPISODES OF MYOCARDIAL ISCHEMIA

The prevalence of this type of finding is unknown, but may include most anginal patients. In these patients, the factors that normally determine the decision to perform or not to perform

Table 2 Distribution of Coronary Artery Disease in Clinical Subsets of Postinfarction Patients

Distribution of Coronary Artery Disease	Timing of Angiography			Clinical Convalescence		Infarction Site			Extent of Infarction	
	Early	Late	Total	Complicated	Uncomplicated	Anterior	Inferior	Indeterminate	Nontransmural	Transmural
Left main	10(11)	0(0)	10(8.5)	6(11)	4(7)	3(5)	7(14)	0(0)	1(4)	9(10)
3 vessels	28(30)	13(52)	41(35)	22(39)	19(31)	27(41)	14(29)	0(0)	10(44)	31(33)
2 vessels	29(32)	8(32)	37(31.5)	15(27)	22(36)	17(26)	18(37)	2(67)	6(26)	31(33)
1 vessel	23(25)	4(16)	27(23)	12(22)	15(25)	17(26)	9(18)	1(33)	5(22)	22(23)
0 vessels	2(2)	0(0)	2(2)	1(1)	1(1)	1(2)	1(2)	0(0)	1(4)	1(1)
Total	92(100)	25(100)	117(100)	56(100)	61(100)	65(100)	49(100)	3(100)	23(100)	94(100)

Percentages are shown in parentheses.
(From J. D. Turner, W. J. Rogers, J. A. Mantel, C. E. Rackley, and R. O. Russell, Jr. *Chest*, 77:58, 1980.)

coronary arteriography — refractoriness of symptoms, degree of abnormality of noninvasive tests — continue to be of prime importance. We have not yet reached the point where consideration of the *total* number of ischemic episodes (symptomatic and silent) is a determining factor in recommending both coronary arteriography and more aggressive management, but perhaps it is not too far off [13].

IV. CORONARY ARTERY DISEASE WITH AND WITHOUT SYMPTOMS: ARE THERE DISTINCTIVE ARTERIOGRAPHIC FEATURES?

One of the more intriguing questions concerning the pathophysiology of silent myocardial ischemia is whether there are any distinctive arteriographic features that help to identify patients with this phenomenon, or with silent myocardial infarction. Accordingly, pertinent date acquired in a number of studies will be reviewed.

Comparisons between *totally asymptomatic* Air Force personnel and angiographically normal persons are provided by Uhl et al. [14]. The distribution of vessel disease in these patients is usually similar to that found in the symptomatic population. For example, Uhl reported that of the 65 men in his study, 32 had one-vessel disease, 17 had two-vessel disease and 16 had three-vessel disease. On the other hand, Kent et al. [5] reported a preponderance of multivessel disease: 41/147 (28%) with one-vessel disaese, 45/147 (31%) with two-vessel disease and 61/147 (41%) with triple-vessel disease. The distribution of standard risk factors was similar to what one expects in a symptomatic coronary artery disease population.

What of patients who are *asymptomatic following a myocardial infarction?* The study from the Duke-Harvard Collaborative Coronary Artery Disease Data Bank [15] can be used as a model for this kind of study since most of the patients had experienced a myocardial infarction. The clinical and angiographic findings in the 171 study patients (127 with and 44 without angina) were comparable. As we noted earlier in this chapter, Turner et al. [6], in a study of 92 asymptomatic postmyocardial infarction patients, found a 35% frequency of triple-vessel disease, 31.5% two-vessel disease and 23% one-vessel disease. Mautner et al. [8] found a similar distribution (Table 1).

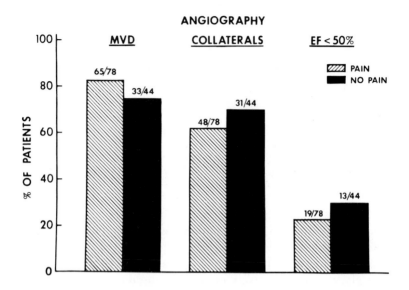

Figure 3   Frequency of multivessel disease (MVD), collateral vessels, and poor ventricular function in patients with and without anginal pain. EF = ejection fraction. (From H. E. Lindsey, Jr., and P. F. Cohn. *Am. Heart J.*, *95*:441, 1978.)

The final group to consider is patients with episodes of *both symptomatic and asymptomatic myocardial ischemia.* Samek et al. [16] studied 102 patients with anginal histories but without angina on a positive exercise test. Thirty-five percent had one-vessel disease, 32% two-vessel disease and 43% three-vessel disease. Lindsey and I [17] also found multivessel disease in 75% of our patients in an earlier, similar study. This compared to 83% (pNS) in patients who were symptomatic during a positive test. The prevalence of collateralization and low ejection fractions was also similar (Figure 3).

Finally, let us consider pateints with *silent myocardial infarctions.* Compared to patients with recognized myocardial infarctions, patients with clinically unrecognized myocardial infarctions have a similar extent of coronary artery disease, as determined by Gohlke et al. [18]. This is the same conclusion that Cabin and Roberts [19] reached in their autopsy study, which was discussed at greater length in Chapter 6.

In conclusion, it appears that there are no striking arteriographic differences between coronary artery disease patients with and without angina.

V. CORONARY ARTERIOGRAPHIC ASSESSMENT OF DIABETICS BEING EVALUATED FOR RENAL TRANSPLANTATION

Because athersclerotic cardiovascular disease is the most common cause of death in diabetic patients with severe renal disease, it has become accepted policy in many hospitals to clarify surgical risk by "screening" diabetic patients with noninvasive tests and/or cardiac catheterization. The findings are often quite dramatic. For example, Bennett et al. found severe coronary artery disease in all such patients in their study [20] (Table 3), while Reinwauch et al. [21] found severe coronary artery disease in 9 of 21 patients.

VI. CONCLUSIONS

Aside from treatment of asymptomatic persons, there is probably no more controversial area than indications for cardiac catheterization in totally asymptomatic individuals. Patients with positive exercise tests — generally those with early onset of ST changes and hypotension or those confirmed by abnormal radionuclide studies — deserve aggressive follow-up with cardiac catheterization. Asymptomatic postinfarction patients with similar findings merit an equally aggressive approach, but this is less of an issue. Results of cardiac catheterization studies do not seem to indicate any particular angiographic patterns in asymptomatic persons with coronary artery disease compared to symptomatic ones.

Table 3   Cardiologic and Lipid Studies in 11 Diabetic Patients with

Case No.	Left Ventricular End-Diastolic Pressure (mmHg)	Ejection Fraction	Coronary Angiography		
			Left Anterior Descending	Right Coronary	Circumflex
1	12	0.66	Minimal, diffuse	Minimal, diffuse	Minimal, diffuse
2	20	0.72	Minimal, diffuse; 30% stenosis	Normal	Normal
3	9	0.72	Minimal, diffuse	Normal	Minimal, diffuse
4	10	0.55	Minimal, diffuse	Minimal, diffuse	Minimal, diffuse
5	5	0.69	75% stenosis	75% stenosis	30% stenosis
6	6	0.81	50% stenosis	Normal	50% stenosis
7	24	0.51	50% stenosis	70% stenosis	50% stenosis
8	15	0.76	60% stenosis	60% stenosis	50% stenosis
9	15	0.59	80% stenosis	Occluded	Moderate diffuse involvement
10	14	0.65	10% stenosis	Minimal, diffuse	20% stenosis
11	15	0.64	70% stenosis	60% stenosis	Minimal diffuse involvement

(From W. M. Bennett, F. Kloster, J. Rosch, J. Barry, and G. A. Porter *Am. J. Med.*, *65*:779, 1978.)

End-Stage Renal Disease

Cholesterol (mg/100 ml)	Triglycerides (mg/100 ml)	Stress Electro-cardiography	Echocardiogram
173	465	Inadequate rate due to fatigue	Left ventricular hypertrophy
192	304	Inadequate rate due to fatigue	Minimal pericardial effusion
219	382	—	Left ventricular hypertrophy
202	226	—	—
207	277	Positive	Left ventricular hypertrophy
162	129	—	Reduced left ventricular compliance
130	90	Inadequate rate due to fatigue	Moderate pericardial effusion, left ventricular hypertrophy
269	200	Positive	Reduced left ventricular compliance
242	196	Positive	Left atrial enlargement
—	—	—	—
424	208	Positive	Left ventricular hypertrophy

REFERENCES

1. J. A. Ambrose. Unsettled indications for coronary angiography. *J. Am. Coll. Cardiol.*, *3*:1575 (1984).
2. C. R. Conti. Detection and management of the asymptomatic patient with coronary artery disease. *Adv. Cardiol.*, *27*:181 (1980).
3. A. Selzer and K. Cohn. Asymptomatic coronary artery disease and coronary bypass surgery. *Am. J. Cardiol.*, *39*:614 (1977).
4. S. E. Epstein. Implications of probability analysis on the strategy used for noninvasive detection of coronary artery disease: Role of single or combined use of exercise electrocardiographic testing, radionuclide cineangiography and myocardial perfusion imaging. *Am. J. Cardiol.*, *46*:491 (1980).
5. K. M. Kent, D. R. Rosing, C. J. Ewels, L. Lipson, R. Bonow, and S. E. Epstein. Prognosis of asymptomatic or mildly symptomatic patients with coronary artery disease. *Am. J. Cardiol.*, *49*:1823 (1982).
6. S. E. Epstein, S. T. Palmeri, and R. E. Patterson. Evaluation of patients after acute myocardial infarction. *N. Engl. J. Med.*, *307*:1487 (1982).
7. Th. W. G. Veenbrink, T. Van Der Werf, P. W. Westerhof, E. O. Robles de Medina, and F. L. Meijler. Is there an indication for coronary angiography in patients under 60 years of age with no or minimal angina pectoris after a first myocardial infarction? *Br. Heart J.*, *53*:30 (1985).
8. R. K. Mautner and J. H. Phillips. Coronary angiography post first myocardial infarction in the asymptomatic or mildly symptomatic patient: Clinical, angiographic, and prospective observations. *Cath. Cardiovasc. Diag.*, 7:1 (1981).
9. B. R. Chaitman, D. Waters, F. Corbara, and M. Bourassa. Predictors of multivessel disease after inferior myocardial infarction. *Circulation, 57*:1085 (1978).
10. R. Miller, A. N. DeMaria, L. A. Vismara, et al.: Chronic stable inferior myocardial infarction: unsuspected harbinger of high risk proximal left coronary arterial obstruction amenable to surgical revascularization. *Am. J. Cardiol.*, *39*:953 (1977).
11. J. D. Turner, W. J. Rogers, J. A. Mantle, C. E. Rackley, and R. O. Russell, Jr. Coronary angiography soon after myocardial infarction. *Chest*, 77:58 (1980).

12. S. H. Rahimtoola. Coronary arteriography in asymptomatic patients after myocardial infarction: The need to distinguish between clinical investigation and clinical care. *Chest*, *77*:53 (1977).

13. P. F. Cohn. Time for a new approach to patients with both symptomatic and asymptomatic episodes of silent myocardial ischemia. *Am. J. Cardiol.*, *54*:1358 (1984).

14. G. S. Uhl and V. Froelicher. Screening for asymptomatic coronary artery disease. *J. Am. Coll. Cardiol.*, *1*:946 (1983).

15. P. F. Cohn, P. Harris, W. H. Barry, R. A. Rosati, P. Rosenbaum, and C. Waternaux. Prognostic importance of anginal symptoms in angiographically defined coronary artery disease. *Am. J. Cardiol.*, *47*:233 (1981).

16. L. Samek, P. Beta, and H. Roskamm. ST-segment depression during exercise without angina pectoris in postinfarction patients: Angiographic findings and prognostic relevance. In *Silent Myocardial Ischemia* (W. Rutishauser and H. Roskamm, eds.), Springer-Verlag, Berlin, 1984, pp. 170–175.

17. H. E. Lindsey, Jr., and P. F. Cohn. "Silent" myocardial ischemia during and after exercise testing in patients with coronary artery disease. *Am. Heart J.*, *95*:441 (1978).

18. H. Gohlke, K. Peters, P. Betz, P. Sturzenhofecker, E. Steinmann, T. Vellguth, and H. Roskamm. Angiography in patients with silent myocardial infarction. In *Silent Myocardial Ischemia* (W. Rutihauser and H. Roskamm, eds.), Springer-Verlag, Berlin, 1984, pp. 138–143.

19. H. S. Cabin and W. C. Roberts. Quantitative comparison of extent of coronary narrowing and size of healed myocardial infarct in 33 necropsy patients with clinically unrecognized ("silent") previous acute myocardial infarction. *Am. J. Cardiol.*, *50*:677 (1982).

20. W. M. Bennett, F. Kloster, J. Rosch, J. Barry, and G. A. Porter. Natural history of asymptomatic coronary arteriographic lesions in diabetic patients with end-stage renal disease. *Am. J. Med.*, *65*:779 (1978).

21. L. Weinrauch, J. A. D'Elia, R. W. Healy, R. E. Gleason, A. R. Christlieb, and O. S. Leland, Jr. Asymptomatic coronary artery disease: Angiographic assessment of diabetics evaluated for renal transplantation. *Circulation*, *58*:1184 (1978).

IV
PROGNOSIS IN ASYMPTOMATIC CORONARY ARTERY DISEASE

12
Prognosis in Patients with Silent Myocardial Ischemia

As we have discussed previously, there are three types of patients with silent myocardial ischemia. One group consists of individuals who have never had symptoms, the second group consists of individuals who are asymptomatic following a myocardial infarction

but still manifest ischemia and the third group includes individuals
who are symptomatic with some of their ischemic episodes but not
with others.

I. PROGNOSIS IN TOTALLY ASYMPTOMATIC INDIVIDUALS

Data in this group of individuals (who have angiographically confirmed disease) is especially hard to come by, since physicians are
naturally reluctant to submit asymptomatic individuals to a potentially dangerous invasive procedure. One of the few surveys that
have provided a large series of subjects is that conducted by the
U.S. Air Force School of Aerospace Medicine in San Antonio,
Texas. This survey was begun by Froelicher and colleagues in the
mid-1970s [1]. Cardiac catheterization was performed on asymptomatic airmen with abnormal treadmill tests, as described in
Chapters 9 and 10. Subsequent treadmill or radionuclide studies,
or both, performed by Froelicher et al. [2] and later by Uhl et al.
[3] resulted in a total of 78 asymptomatic airmen with significant
coronary artery disease being detected. Along with 12 other airmen with minimal coronary artery disease, this group was followed
for several years to evaluate those factors influencing prognosis.

In the most recent report from the San Antonio survey, Hickman et al. [4] reported that 22 of the 78 airmen with significant
disease (more than 50% luminal stenosis) developed overt signs of
coronary artery disease, i.e., angina, myocardial infarction, death
within a 4-90-month follow-up period. The mean time was 57
months and the men ranged in age from 47 to 54 years. Of the 22
with significant coronary artery disease, 16 developed angina at a
mean duration of 31.5 months, four sustained a myocardial infarction and two died suddenly. In addition to the 22, six other men
developed symptoms at a later time (mean age 46 months). Of
these six, five developed angina and one died suddenly. The authors
investigated the influence of the four standard coronary risk factors
(cigarette smoking, hyperlipidemia, diabetes and hypertension) and
found that at least three of these risk factors were present in nearly
half of the men who had subsequent cardiac events. These provoca-
tive findings highlight the importance of risk factors in prognosis of
asymptomatic men, as well as in the screening of such populations,
as discussed in Section III.

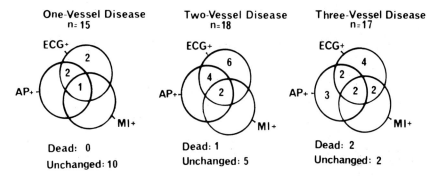

Figure 1 Venn diagrams showing the relation between baseline angiographic findings and coronary artery disease (CAD) events during a mean follow-up of 8 1/2 years in 50 men with asymptomatic CAD. AP = angina pectoris. (From J. Erikssen and E. Thaulow. In *Silent Myocardial Ischemia* [W. Rutishauser and H. Roskamm, eds.], Springer–Verlag, Berlin, 1984, pp. 156–164.)

In the smaller series reported by Langou et al. [5] from Yale University, the authors followed their 12 subjects with significant coronary artery disease for three years. In that period of time, three men developed angina and one a myocardial infarction, though none died.

The most ambitious of all of these studies was the one performed in Norway by Erikssen and colleagues [6]. From a large cohort of men aged 40–59 years who underwent a comprehensive cardiovascular screening in 1972–75, 69 were identified as having significant coronary artery disease, 18 with one-vessel disease, 25 with two-vessel disease and 26 with three-vessel disease. Fifty of the sixty-nine men were unequivocally felt to have asymptomatic coronary artery disease; in the other 19, it was questionable whether mild symptoms were present. After an eight-to-ten-year period of following the 50 asymptomatic men, the authors found that three died from cardiac disease and seven had a myocardial infarction (five of which were silent) [7, 8]. In addition, as depicted in Figure 1, 16 other men developed angina pectoris. Twenty-four patients had repeat angiograms; 23 of the 24 had progression (56%) (Figure 2) and 11 underwent coronary bypass surgery. Thus, a total of 28 (56%) either died, had a myocardial infarction, devel-

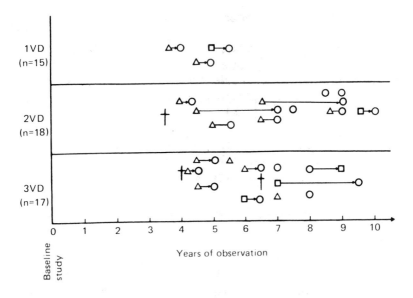

Figure 2   CAD progression in relation to baseline coronary angiographic findings and years of follow-up in 50 men with asymptomatic CAD diagnosed at the baseline study. Arrow length indicates the interval between first CAD event and coronary angiographic verification of CAD progression. † = death; o = angiographic progression; □ = myocardial infarction; △ = AP. (From J. Erikssen and E. Thaulow. In *Silent Myocardial Ischemia* [W. Rutishauser and H. Roskamm, eds.], Springer-Verlag, Berlin, 1984, pp. 156–164.)

oped angina or had progression on coronary angiography. (Men with and without these events were of similar age, had similar heart rates and blood pressure.) The total mortality was less than 1%/year, but this may be skewered by the 11 men sent for bypass surgery. Clinical events were observed mostly in men with multivessel disease. The authors concluded that once they are diagnosed, subjects with asymptomatic coronary artery disease should be followed yearly. In that manner, rapid detection of clinical events is possible and appropriate therapy can be initiated. This is usually conservative, though the authors infer that patients with left main disease — like their symptomatic counterparts — should be offered aggressive management in light of the "malignant" course of the five patients in the study — two dead and three others with angiographic or clinical progression.

Another interesting subgroup of asymptomatic patients are those with diabetes mellitus and end-stage renal disease who are being considered for transplantation. Bennett et al. [9] reported on 11 consecutive patients (previously discussed in Chapter 11), eight of whom died within the 20-month mean follow-up period; six died of cardiac causes (Table 1).

In the nonangiographic group, several epidemiologic studies have called attention to the increased mortality associated with positive exercise tests in asymptomatic persons (see Chapter 9).

II. PROGNOSIS IN PATIENTS WHO ARE ASYMPTOMATIC FOLLOWING A MYOCARDIAL INFARCTION

These studies usually have heterogeneous populations. For example, an investigation at the National Institutes of Health followed 20 patients who were asymptomatic after an infarction but included five other totally asymptomatic persons and 122 mildly asymptomatic persons (61 of whom had prior infarctions) in their study group [10]. As expected, there was a high frequency of coronary risk factors in this group. Thus, 90 patients were (or had been) cigarette smokers, 33 had hypertension, 22 had hypercholesterolemia and 48 had either clinical diabetes or an abnormal glucose tolerance test. Forty-one of the patients had single-vessel coronary artery disease (28%), 45 had double-vessel disease (31%) and 61 had triple-vessel disease (41%). In the entire group, the authors could not find any combination of *clinical* risk factors that identified a high-risk subgroup, and the entire group mortality was 3%/year, a figure lower than reported for symptomatic groups. The life table analysis of the entire cohort of 147 patients is depicted in Figure 3. In the four years of follow-up, eight deaths occurred. The triple-vessel group was studied separately. Figure 4 shows that patients with good exercise capacity had an annual mortality of 4%, while those with poor exercise capacity had an annual mortality of 9%; total mortality was 6%. Combined attrition (mortality plus progression of symptoms) was also better in the patients with triple-vessel disease and good exercise tolerance, but this difference did not achieve statistical significance (Figure 5). In a follow-up study, the authors evaluated only patients with resting

Table 1   Clinical Course of Asymptomatic Diabetic Patients with Coronary Arteriographic Abnormalities

Case No.	Duration of Follow-up to Death or to Present Analysis (mo)	Modality of Renal Disease Treatment	Outcome of Therapy	Pathology	Worsening of Hyperlipoproteinemia	Comments
1	30	Rejection of two cadaver transplants	Alive on dialysis	—	Yes	—
2	18	Cadaver transplant	Death from stroke	Diffuse coronary arteriosclerosis	No	Normal renal function at time of death
3	7	Live donor transplant	Death from sepsis and cardiac arrest	No necropsy	No	Normal renal function at time of death
4	12	Long-term hemodialysis	Death while on machine	No necropsy	Yes	History of chest pain and drop in blood pressure prior to death
5	38	Long-term dialysis	Alive	—	No	Angina pectoris when hematocrit less than 25%

6	28	Long-term dialysis	Death from myocardial infarct	Extensive coronary disease, fresh infarct	No	Infarct 6 hours after dialysis treatment
7	36	Related donor transplant	Alive	—	No	Angina pectoris for 6 mo. hypertension and decreased graft function due to graft arteriosclerosis
8	18	Long-term dialysis	Death from infarct and pulmonary edema	No necropsy	Yes	—
9	4	Long-term dialysis	Death from massive myocardial infarct	No necropsy	No	Major gastrointestinal hemorrhage preceded fatal event
10	11	Cadaver transplant	Death from myocardial infarct	Confirmed coronary disease postmortem	No	Rejection, uremic pericarditis preceded fatal event
11	16	Long-term dialysis	Death following coronary vein bypass surgery	Fresh myocardial infarct	Yes	Disabling angina; marked progression demonstrated on preoperative angiogram

(From W. B. Bennett, F. Kloster, J. Rosch, J. Barry, and G. A. Porter. *Am. J. Med.,* 65:779, 1979.)

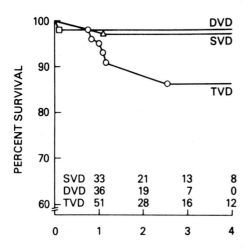

Figure 3   Life table analysis of 147 patients with single- (SVD), double- (DVD) and triple-vessel (TVD) coronary artery disease for up to four years after entry into the study. Eight deaths occurred during the follow-up period at which time the probability data were generated. The line is extended to four years in each group after the last death occurred, although this is an extrapolation and not based on another set of probability data. The number of patients in the study at each yearly interval in each subgroup are shown at bottom. (From K. M. Kent, D. R. Rosing, C. J. Ewels, L. Lipson, R. Bonow, and S. E. Epstein. *Am. J. Cardiol.*, *49*:1823, 1982.)

ejection fractions > 0.40 (new patients with ejection fractions > 0.40 were also added). The purpose of the new study of 117 patients was "to test the hypothesis that in patients with preserved left ventricular function at rest, the presence and severity of reversible ischemia (measured by both radionuclide angiography and exercise electrocardiography) may be a more specific predictor of prognosis during medical therapy." The authors found that patients with three-vessel disease, positive ST segment response to exercise, exercise capacity less than 120 watts and an exercise-induced fall in ejection fraction had an annual mortality rate of 7% [11], confirming their hypothesis. We will discuss these mortality figures again in Section V when we contrast them with the results

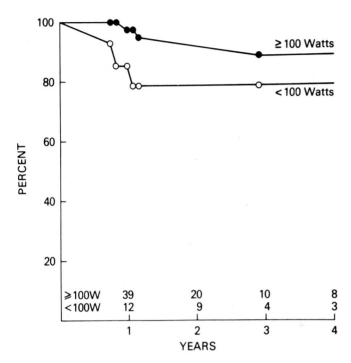

Figure 4   Life table analysis comparing patients with triple-vessel disease who were able to achieve 100 or more watts on the bicycle ergometer and patients who had poor exercise capacity (less than 100 watts). In this comparison between two groups, probability data are calculated for both groups when an event occurs in either group. (From K. M. Kent, D. R. Rosing, C. J. Ewels, L. Lipson, R. Bonow, and S. E. Epstein. *Am. J. Cardiol.*, *49*:1823, 1982.)

of medically treated patients from the Coronary Artery Surgical Study (CASS) registry.

Another study from the Duke-Harvard Collaborative Coronary Artery Disease Data Bank also included a mixture of totally asymptomatic and partially symptomatic patients with angiographically documented coronary artery disease who had no angina symptoms for at least several months prior to coronary angiography and who were not taking antianginal medications nor had undergone coro-

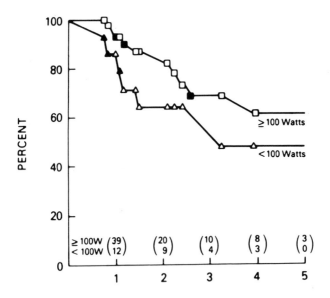

Figure 5   Probability that patients with triple-vessel disease will survive and remain in symptomatically stable condition for 48 months as assessed by exercise capacity at the initial evaluation. ■▲ = death, □△ = positive symptoms. (From K. M. Kent, D. R. Rosing, C. J. Ewels, L. Lipson, R. Bonow, and S. E. Epstein. *Am. J. Cardiol.*, *49*:1823, 1982.)

nary bypass surgery. Thirty-two had prior infarctions. The 44 patients were matched with 127 symptomatic patients from the same data bank. The computerized matching process was based on five variables that reflected coronary anatomy and left ventricular function. Originally we had hoped to match each of the 44 asymptomatic patients with three symptomatic patients to ensure a large enough data base, but this was not always possible; hence, the final figure for the control group was 127 rather than 132. In addition to the five variables noted earlier, we also compared the frequency of other variables once the groups were selected by the computer. This was to insure that the results of the survival analysis were not influenced by descriptors that were not selected to be matched by the computer. This comparison is depicted in Table 2;

Table 2   Clinical and Angiographic Findings in Study Patients
With and Without Anginal Symptoms

	Without Anginal Symptoms (n = 44)	With Anginal Symptoms (n = 127)
Mean age	47.6	49.0
Male sex	41 (93%)	107 (84%)
Diabetes	2 (4%)	8 (6%)
Hypertension	13 (29%)	27 (21%)
Diagnostic Q waves in electrocardiogram	23 (53%)	76 (60%)
Positive exercise test	17/31 (55%)	48/96 (50%)
Two vessel disease	13 (30%)	38 (30%)
Three vessel disease	18 (40%)	51 (40%)
Left main coronary arterial stenosis	0	0
Left anterior descending arterial stenosis	36 (82%)	91 (72%)
Totally occluded vessels	12 (27%)	34 (27%)
Abnormal left ventricular contraction pattern	32 (73%)	95 (75%)
Left ventricular end-diastolic pressure > 18 mm Hg	8 (18%)	18 (14%)
Arteriovenous oxygen difference > 5.5 volumes percent	9 (21%)	23 (18%)

(From P. F. Cohn, P. Harris, W. H. Barry, R. A. Rosati, P. Rosenbaum, and C. Waternaux. *Am. J. Cardiol.*, 47:233, 1981.)

there were no significant differences between the two groups. Survival curves in the entire group are shown in Figure 6. Mean follow-up time was 3 1/2 years. There was an 81% survival rate for the total asymptomatic group at seven years (yearly mortality 2.7%), compared with a 62% survival rate for the symptomatic group (yearly mortality 5.4%). The worst prognosis was in the subgroup with three-vessel disease (4.7% vs. 8.7% in the symptomatic group) (Figure 7). Two of the four patients in the sympto-

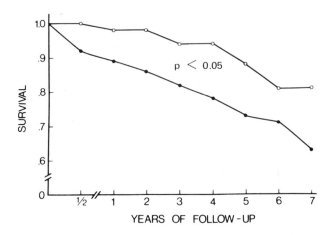

Figure 6   Survival curves for 44 patients without anginal symptoms (○) and 127 matched patients with anginal symptoms (●),
in the Duke-Harvard Coronary Artery Disease (CAD) Data Bank.
(From P. F. Cohn, P. Harris, W. H. Barry, R. A. Rosati, P. Rosenbaum, and C. Waternaux. *Am. J. Cardiol.*, *47*:233, 1981.)

matic group who died had anginal symptoms at least six months
before their death; development of anginal symptoms eventually
was reported in 30% of the patients by the end of the four-year
follow-up.

   In addition to these studies, there are numerous reports des-
cribing prognosis in patients who have sustained an acute myocardial infarction. Short-term survival statistics based on the postinfarction exercise studies indicate that exercise-induced ST segment depression markedly increases the one-year mortality. In
some of these studies, prognosis in those patients who were
asymptomatic and had positive exercise tests denoting active,
though silent, myocardial ischemia could be gleaned from the raw
data. For example, in the study by Theroux et al. [13], 210 patients who had no ᴜvert heart failure and had been free of chest
pain for at least four days were exercised one day before discharge
from the hospital. The one-year mortality rate was 2.1% (3 of 146)
in patients without ischemic ST changes during exercise and 27%

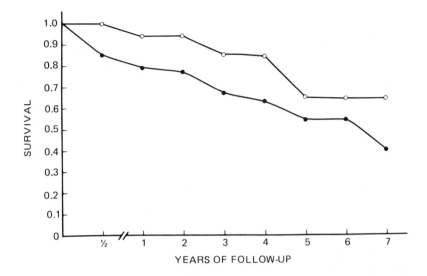

Figure 7 Survival curves for 17 patients (○) with three-vessel coronary artery disease but without anginal symptoms compared to 49 patients (●) with three-vessel disease and anginal symptoms, in the Duke-Harvard Coronary Artery Disease (CAD) Data Bank.

(17 of 64) in those with such changes ($p < 0.001$). The authors reported that angina in the presence of ST segment depression had no effect on these statistics. Thus, 10 of 37 patients with ST depression on the exercise test but without angina died, compared with 7 of 27 with both exercise-induced ST depression and angina. More recently, Gibson and Beller [14] have reported that postinfarction patients at highest risk are those with thallium-201 redistribution defects.

Other prognostic studies involving therapy are discussed in Section V.

III. PROGNOSIS IN PATIENTS WITH BOTH SYMPTOMATIC AND ASYMPTOMATIC ISCHEMIC EPISODES

Several studies have investigated the prognosis of patients with effort-angina who have a positive exercise test without angina. Presumably, these individuals have both symptomatic and silent

ischemic episodes during daily activities. Rabaeus et al. [15] studied
150 such patients with coronary artery disease, 40 with a prior
infarction but no cardiac catheterization and 110 who were cathe-
terized. Forty-three patients had one-vessel disease, 37 had two-
vessel disease and 30 had three-vessel disease. Mean follow-up time
was 45 months. Major coronary events (unstable angina, myocardial infarction, coronary artery bypass surgery or sudden death)
occurred in 76 patients (51%). These events were significantly
associated with extent of coronary artery disease. When correlations with other factors during the exercise test were made between
these 76 patients and the 74 without major coronary events, no
positive relationship was noted.

Samek et al. [16] studied 102 patients post infarction (23 with
one-vessel disease, 31 with two-vessel disease and 48 with three-
vessel disease). The five-year mortality rate in 72 medically treated
patients was 7% and the rate of cardiac events (death or nonfatal
myocardial infarction) was 12%. Samek et al. compared these
figures to those of a larger group of 325 patients with both ischemic changes and angina during testing. Mortality in this symptomatic control group was 16% and the rate of cardiac events 21%.
The authors concluded that prognosis was better in patients *without*
angina during positive exercise tests. Rabaeus et al. had no such
control group.

When follow-up results in patients subjected to long-term ambulatory monitoring (as described in Chapter 8) are available, we can
expect even more pertinent data on this subject to emerge. An example of this type of study has been provided — in preliminary form
[17] — by Nademanee et al. They studied 72 patients with unstable angina. Fifteen medically controlled patients had Holter
monitoring that revealed more than 60 minutes of silent ischemic
episodes in a 24-hour period. Within 6 months, two patients had
died, three others had nonfatal infarctions and the other nine required semiurgent surgery for increasing symptoms. The authors
concluded that "persistent silent myocardial ischemia is an index
of serious prognosis" in patients with unstable angina.

IV. CONCLUSIONS

In general, prognosis in totally asymptomatic individuals appears
better than in symptomatic persons. However, in studies in which

totally asymptomatic patients and patients who are asymptomatic after an infarction (and in some instances, mildly asymptomatic patients) are reviewed, there appears to be a subgroup of individuals with three-vessel disease who have far from a benign prognosis. Mortality in this group ranges from 4 to 9%, depending on the selection criteria used. What effect the presence of frequent silent ischemic episodes have on the prognosis of patients with angina is still unresolved.

REFERENCES

1. V. F. Froelicher, A. J. Thompson, M. R. Longo, J. Triebwasser, and M. C. Lancaster. Value of exercise testing for screening asymptomatic men for latent coronary heart disease. *Prog. Cardiovasc. Dis.*, *18*:265 (1976).
2. G. S. Uhl and V. Froelicher. Screening for asymptomatic coronary artery disease. *J. Am. Coll. Cardiol.*, *1*:946 (1983).
3. G. S. Uhl, T. N. Kay, and J. R. Hickman, Jr. Comparison of exercise radionuclide angiography and thallium perfusion imaging in detecting coronary disease in asymptomatic men. *J. Cardiac Rehabil.*, *2*:118 (1982).
4. J. R. Hickman, Jr., G. S. Uhl, R. L. Cook, P. J. Engel, and A. Hopkirk. A natural history study of asymptomatic coronary disease (abstr). *Am. J. Cardiol.*, *45*:422 (1980).
5. R. A. Langou, E. K. Huang, M. J. Kelley, and L. S. Cohen. Predictive accuracy of coronary artery calcification and abnormal exercise test for coronary artery disease in asymptomatic men. *Circulation*, *62*:1196 (1980).
6. J. Erikssen, I. Enge, K. Forfang, and O. Storstein. False positive diagnostic tests and coronary angiographic findings in 105 presumably healthy males. *Circulation*, *54*:371 (1976).
7. J. Erikssen and E. Thaulow. Follow-up of patients with asymptomatic myocardial ischemia. In *Silent Myocardial Ischemia* (W. Rutishauser and H. Roskamm, eds.), Springer-Verlag, Berlin, 1984, pp. 156–164.
8. J. Erikssen and R. Mundal. The patient with coronary disease without infarction: Can a high risk group be identified? *Ann. NY Acad. Sci.*, *382*:438 (1982).
9. W. M. Bennett, F. Kloster, J. Rosch, J. Barry and G. A. Porter. Natural history of asymptomatic coronary arteriographic lesions

    in diabetic patients with end-stage renal disease. *Am. J. Med.*,
    65:779–784 (1978).
10. K. M. Kent, D. R. Rosing, C. J. Ewels, L. Lipson, R. Bonow,
    and S. E. Epstein. Prognosis of asymptomatic or mildly symp-
    tomatic patients with coronary artery disease. *Am. J. Cardiol.*,
    49:1823 (1982).
11. R. O. Bonow, K. M. Kent, D. R. Rosing, K. K. G. Lan, E.
    Lakatos, J. S. Borer, S. L. Bacharach, M. V. Green, and S. E.
    Epstein. Exercise-induced ischemia in mildly symptomatic
    patients with coronary-artery disease and preserved left ven-
    tricular function: Identification of subgroups at risk of death
    during medical therapy. *N. Engl. J. Med.*, *311*:1339 (1984).
12. P. F. Cohn, P. Harris, W. H. Barry, R. A. Rosati, P. Rosenbaum,
    and C. Waternaux. Prognostic importance of anginal symp-
    toms in angiographically defined coronary artery disease. *Am.
    J. Cardiol.*, *47*:233 (1981).
13. P. Theroux, D. D. Waters, C. Halphen, J. C. Debaisieux, and
    H. F. Mizgala. Prognostic value of exercise testing soon after
    myocardial infarction. *N. Engl. J. Med.*, *301*:341 (1979).
14. R. S. Gibson and G. A. Beller. Prevalence and significance
    of exercise-induced painless ST segment depression two
    weeks post infarction (abstr). *Circulation*, *70*(Suppl II):
    II–60 (1984).
15. M. Rabaeus, A. Righetti, and P. Moret. Long-term follow-up
    of patients with positive exercise test without angina in a
    referred population. In *Silent Myocardial Ischemia* (W. Ruti-
    shauser and H. Roskamm, eds.), Springer–Verlag, Berlin,
    1984, pp. 165–169.
16. L. Samek, P. Betz, and H. Roskamm. ST-segment depression
    during exercise without angina pectoris in postinfarction
    patients: Angiographic findings and prognostic relevance.
    In *Silent Myocardial Ischemia* (W. Rutishauser and H. Ros-
    kamm, eds.), Springer–Verlag, Berlin, 1984, pp. 170–175.
17. K. Nademanee, V. Intarachot, M. Plontek, F. Vaghalwalla-
    mody, D. Reider, M. Josephson, and B. N. Singh. Silent
    myocardial ischemia on Holter: Has it clinical or prognostic
    significance? (abstr). *Circulation*, *70* (Suppl 11):11–451
    (1984).

13
Relation of Silent Myocardial Ischemia to Sudden Death, Silent Myocardial Infarction and Ischemic Cardiomyopathy

In addition to the overall prognostic picture provided in Chapter 12, there are three potential complications of silent myocardial ischemia that warrant special comment.

I. SILENT MYOCARDIAL ISCHEMIA AND SUDDEN DEATH

Sudden death is often defined as death occurring within hours of collapse, etc. in a person with or without prior overt cardiac disease in whom there is no other probable cause of death. In witnessed deaths (in-hospital or out-of-hospital) the most common arrhythmia is ventricular fibrillation [1].

Sudden death represents a major source of cardiovascular mortality in the United States. It has been estimated that some 300,000 persons die in this manner every year [2]. Most have coronary artery disease and many have not had *any* prior clinical evidence of heart disease.

The Framingham study has analyzed the risk factors for this phenomenon in 5209 persons and found that the "classical" risk factors of coronary artery disease appear to be risk factors for sudden death as well, especially in men [2]. Pathologic studies at necropsy have revealed several differences between those patients who were previously asymptomatic compared to those patients who had histories of angina pectoris and/or a clinical acute myocardial infarction [3]. Peak age was 41–60 (Figure 1) and men predominated. There was a higher frequency of left main disease

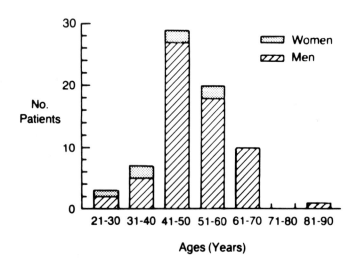

Figure 1   Age distribution in 70 patients with sudden coronary death. (From C. A. Warnes and W. C. Roberts. *Am. J. Cardiol.*, *54*:65, 1984.)

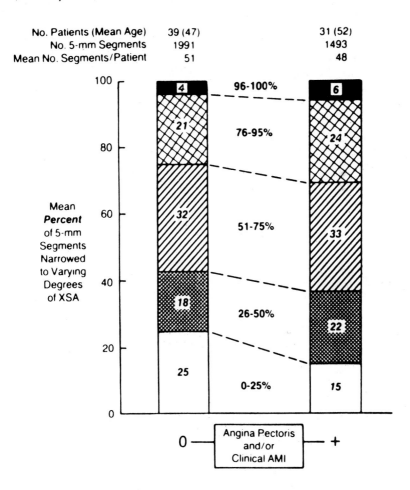

Figure 2   Mean percent of 5-mm segments of the sum of the four major coronary arteries narrowed to varying degrees in cross-sectional area (XSA) in 70 patients with sudden coronary death: comparison of 39 patients without and 31 patients with a clinical acute myocardial infarction (AMI) or angina or both. (From C. A. Warnes and W. C. Roberts. *Am. J. Cardiol.*, *54*:65, 1984.)

and a lower frequency of one-vessel disease in the symptomatic group. Quantitative analysis showed a significantly higher mean percent of severely narrowed segments in the symptomatic group and less minimal narrowing (Figure 2).

The degree of vascular pathology not withstanding, the intriguing question is whether patients with silent myocardial ischemia are as likely — or more likely — to develop sudden death than their symptomatic counterparts. The operational hypothesis is that in the absence of an effective anginal warning system [4], high-risk individuals will continue to exert themselves until catastrophic events (sudden death or myocardial infarction) occur.

It is obvious that the widespread and extensive coronary atherosclerosis present at autopsy in individuals dying suddenly and unexpectedly did not occur overnight (although the final, occluding thrombus — when present — is a sudden event). Few studies have addressed the issue of whether the population with asymptomatic coronary artery disease forms the pool from which a certain number of persons will surface each year as victims of sudden death or nonfatal myocardial infarctions. Preliminary evidence from a study performed at the Hennepin County Medical Center in Minnesota [5] provides some tentative conclusions in this regard. These investigators studied 19 persons who were successfully resuscitated from ventricular fibrillation that took place outside the hospital. All 19 had angiographically confirmed coronary artery disease and 11 of the 19 had no prior history of heart disease. During bicycle exercise testing in the catheterization laboratory, nearly all the patients developed silent myocardial ischemia on their ECGs. Ventriculography also showed painless wall motion abnormalities. The severity of left ventricular dysfunction was similar in asymptomatic compared to previously symptomatic patients. Thus, silent ischemia may play a role in the genesis of sudden death. Two other anecdotal reports showed similar results. Kattus at UCLA (personal communication) studied five previously asymptomatic coronary patients who were resuscitated from sudden death and demonstrated silent ischemia on exercise testing. Myerburg at the University of Miami (personal communication) has had a similar experience with three patients.

A more direct relationship between silent myocardial ischemia and sudden death was reported by Erikksen et al. [6]. In this study, 3 of 50 totally asymptomatic persons died suddenly and unexpectedly. Interestingly, seven others developed myocardial infarctions, of which two were silent. All three of the dead patients and six of the seven patients with myocardial infarctions had multivessel disease.

Table 1 Incidence of SD in Coronary Artery Disease

Patient Category		Annual Incidence (per 1000)
Symptomatic	Stable effort angina	20–27
	Unstable angina	40–60
	Acute myocardial infarction	⩾ 20%
	Previous infarction	50
Asymptomatic	No previous acute myocardial infarction	4.4 [16]
		2.9 [17]
		10 [8, 18]
	Previous myocardial infarction	12 [24]

SD = sudden death. Numbers in brackets indicate references in original article. (From G. A. Feruglio. In *Silent Myocardial Ischemia* [W. Rutishauser and H. Roskmann, eds.], Springer–Verlag, Berlin, 1984.)

In the U.S. Air Force study, Hickman et al. [7] recorded two cases of sudden death (for an annual rate of 4.4/1000), while Feruglio [8] reported rates of 10/1000 in one series and 12/1000 in another series. This compares to rates of 2.9/1000 in epidemiologic studies using positive exercise tests without angiographic confirmation. By contrast, rates of 20–27/1000 for stable angina patients and 40–60/1000 for those with unstable angina have been reported [8] (Table 1).

What implications do these data have in relation to vigorous exercise in asymptomatic individuals? We know there is a small risk of sudden death in persons participating in vigorous sports. Northcote and Ballantyne reviewed the literature and found 109 such instances of which 80 (73%) were attributed to coronary artery disease found at autopsy [9]. They felt medical screening, including exercise testing, might be helpful in identifying some of the individuals at highest risk. By contrast, Malinow et al. found only one case of sudden death in a 10-year retrospective analysis of YMCA sports facilities in the United States [10]. Therefore, they felt it was not important to screen such persons. Recently, Siscovick et al. [11] interviewed the wives of 133 men without known prior heart disease who had suffered a cardiac arrest. They concluded that those persons who engaged in low levels of habitual physical activity had a greater risk of sudden death during vigorous exercise compared to more physically active men. Even though the frequency of these deaths is not common — jogging deaths, for example, are unusual — exercise ECG screening has been advocated prior to performing vigorous activity.

II. SILENT MYOCARDIAL ISCHEMIA AND SILENT MYOCARDIAL INFARCTION

It is tempting to speculate that if myocardial infarction occurs — rather than sudden death — it is more likely to be silent in this group of individuals. Are there any data to support this conjecture? As noted earlier in Erikksen's study [6], 2 of 50 asymptomatic patients with angiographically confirmed disease developed silent infarctions. Other cases have not been reported, though one could speculate that this circumstance must be more common, since 20–25% of all infarctions are silent.

III. SILENT MYOCARDIAL ISCHEMIA AND ISCHEMIC CARDIOMYOPATHY

Ischemia of the myocardium can cause diffuse fibrosis with the resultant clinical syndrome being indistinguishable from that of a primary congestive cardiomyopathy [12]. It has generally been assumed that these cases represent "burnt-out" postinfarction patients who no longer have ischemic foci. A history of angina is usually, but not invariably, present. However, in many cases there has been neither an anginal history nor a history of a symptomatic infarction. Pantely and Bristow [12] speculate that "repeated episodes of silent ischemia, though brief, or silent infarction, though small, may result in congestive ischemic cardiomyopathy" in such patients. Raper et al. [13] in their small series of patients with severe painless ischemia offer dramatic evidence of how a painless episode can lead to marked left ventricular dysfunction, including pulmonary edema.

    Survival in patients with this syndrome — as in all types of cardiomyopathy — is directly related to the degree of left ventricular dysfunction.

IV. CONCLUSIONS

It is intriguing to speculate that silent myocardial ischemia can lead to sudden death, silent infarcts or ischemic cardiomyopathy. There is evidence to confirm this sequence in some patients, but the numbers are too small to permit sweeping generalizations.

REFERENCES

1. S. Goldstein, L. Friedman, R. Hutchinson, P. Canner, D. Romhilt, R. Schlant, R. Sobrino, J. Verter, A. Wasserman, and the Aspirin Myocardial Infarction Study Research Group. Timing, mechanism and clinical setting of witnessed deaths in postmyocardial infarction patients. *J. Am. Coll. Cardiol.*, *3*: 111 (1984).

2. A. Schatzkin, L. A. Cupples, T. Heeren, S. Morelock, M. Mucatel, and W. B. Kannel. The epidemiology of sudden unexpected death: Risk factors for men and women in the Framingham Heart Study. *Am. Heart J.*, *107*:1300 (1984).

3. C. A. Warnes and W. C. Roberts. Sudden coronary death: Relation of amount and distribution of coronary narrowing at necropsy to previous symptoms of myocardial ischemia, left ventricular scarring and heart weight. *Am. J. Cardiol.*, *54*: 65 (1984).

4. P. F. Cohn. Silent myocardial ischemia in patients with a defective anginal warning system. *Am. J. Cardiol.*, *45*:697 (1980).

5. B. Sharma, G. Francis, M. Hodges, and R. Asinger. Demonstration of exercise-induced ischemia without angina in patients who recover from out-of-hospital ventricular fibrillation (abstr). *Am. J. Cardiol.*, *47*:445 (1981).

6. J. Erikssen and E. Thaulow. Follow-up of patients with asymptomatic myocardial ischemia. In *Silent Myocardial Ischemia* (W. Rutishauser and H. Roskamm, eds.), Springer-Verlag, Berlin, 1984, pp. 156–164.

7. J. R. Hickman, Jr., G. S. Uhl, R. L. Cook, P. J. Engel, and A. Hopkirk. A natural study of asymptomatic coronary disease (abstr). *Am. J. Cardiol.*, *45*:422 (1980).

8. G. A. Feruglio. Sudden death in patients with asymptomatic coronary heart disease. In *Silent Myocardial Ischemia* (W.

Rutishauser and H. Roskmann, eds.), Springer–Verlag, Berlin, 1984, pp. 144–150.

9. R. J. Northcote and D. Ballantyne. Sudden cardiac death in sport. *Br. Med. J.*, *287*:1357 (1983).

10. M. R. Malinow, D. L. McGarry, and K. S. Kuehl. Is exercise testing indicated for asymptomatic active people? *J. Cardiac Rehabil.*, *4*:376 (1984).

11. D. S. Siscovick, N. S. Weiss, R. H. Fletcher, and T. Lasky. Relation between vigorous exercise and primary cardiac arrest. *N. Engl. J. Med.*, *311*:874 (1984).

12. G. A. Pantely and J. D. Bristow. Ischemic cardiomyopathy. *Prog. Cardiovasc. Dis.*, *27*:95 (1984).

13. A. J. Raper, A. Hastillo, and W. J. Paulsen. The syndrome of sudden severe painless myocardial ischemia. *Am. Heart J.*, *107*:813 (1984).

14
Prognosis After Silent Myocardial Infarction and Myocardial Infarction Without Preceding Angina

The natural history of coronary artery disease is complex because of the numerous "subsets" of patients with or without angina, with or without infarctions, etc. [1]. Unfortunately, data on prognosis following silent infarctions are sparse. The greatest source of data concerning this subset of patients has been the Framingham Study.

I. SILENT MYOCARDIAL INFARCTION

The Framingham survey was begun in 1948. A standard, thorough, cardiovascular examination was done biennially to detect newly developed cardiovascular disease. In addition, data on cardiovascular endpoints was also obtained by daily surveillance of hospital admission records at Framingham Union Hospital.

As discussed previously in Chapter 5, the myocardial infarctions were designated as "unrecognized" and then further subdivided into atypical or silent, depending on whether the patients — in retrospect — could identify any complaints as having possibly been compatible with an acute myocardial infarction. (About half of the 108 infarctions were of the truly silent type.) As reported in the 20-year follow-up, the three-year mortality rates for both unrecognized and recognized myocardial infarctions were similar [2].

In their most recent report (26-year follow-up), the Framingham investigators have updated their results [3, 4]. As before, there are no data available on prognosis in the immediate convalescent period since, by definition, these patients are not identified until the next routine ECG is performed. However, in those who survived the initial period, the mortality statistics are sobering. As depicted in Figure 1, unrecognized infarctions are as potentially lethal as the symptomatic kind. Sudden deaths occur with some frequency, and at about nine times that seen in the general population. Although less prone to angina (18% vs. 59%) (Table 1), patients with unrecognized infarctions develop congestive heart failure just as often (Table 2). Reinfarction is also common (3%/year in men and 10%/year in women). About 50% of the recurrences are fatal.

In the Israeli study of Medalie et al. [5], the mortality following unrecognized myocardial infarctions was markedly lower than after recognized myocardial infarctions — unlike the Framingham experience.

II. MYOCARDIAL INFARCTION WITHOUT PRECEDING ANGINA

In patients who survive an acute myocardial infarction, half did not have angina pectoris before the infarction [6, 7]. As noted

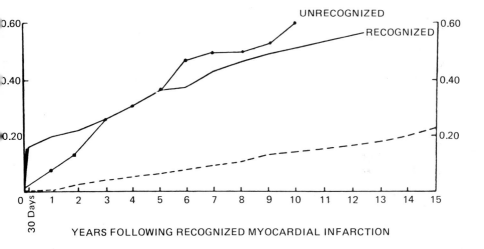

Figure 1   Death following recognized and unrecognized myocardial infarctions (MI) in men of all ages in the Framingham Study. (From W. B. Kannel and R. D. Abbott. In *Silent Myocardial Ischemia* ——— = with MI; — — — = free of MI. [W. Rutishauser and H. Roskamm, eds.], Springer–Verlag, Berlin, 1984, pp. 131–137.)

Table 1   Proportion of ECG-Documented Myocardial Infarctions (MI) Followed by Angina Pectoris (AP) in Subjects Aged 30–62 Years on Entry. Framingham Study, 22-Year Follow-Up

	Number with MI	Followed by AP	
		n	%
Unrecognized	98	18	18
Recognized	190	113	59
Total	288	114	45

Note: 89 patients had prior angina pectoris or died and were eliminated from consideration.
(From W.B. Kannel and R. D. Abbott. In *Silent Myocardial Ischemia* [W. Rutishauser and H. Roskamm, eds.], Springer–Verlag, Berlin, 1984, pp. 131–137.)

Table 2 Proportion of ECG-Documented Myocardial Infarctions
Followed by Cardiac Failure in Subjects 30–62 Years of Age at
Entry. Framingham Study, 22-Year Follow-Up

| | Number | Followed by Cardiac Failure | |
		n	%
Unrecognized	100	21	21
Recognized	221	55	25
Total	321	76	24

(From W. B. Kannel and R. D. Abbott. In *Silent Myocardial Ischemia* [W.
Rutishauser and H. Roskamm, eds.], Springer–Verlag, Berlin, 1984, pp. 131–
137.)

previously in Chapter 5, there is a high association of one-vessel disease (82%) in such patients [8]. One would suspect that prognosis
might, therefore, be better in this type of patient and indeed Midwall et al. [8] reported a lower frequency of postinfarction angina.
Mortality figures were not available. Harper et al. [5] did report on
hospital mortality in their series; it was 12% in patients without
preceding angina compared to 20% in patients with chronic stable
angina. Long-term mortality statistics were also not available in
this study. A recent study by Matsuda et al. [9] suggests that postinfarction left ventricular function is better in patients with angina
and an occluded left anterior descending coronary artery compared
to those without angian. No ready explanation for this finding is
available, though the authors suggest better developed collaterals
may be involved. Cortina et al. [10] reported similar findings.

III. CONCLUSIONS

Silent myocardial infarctions are as potentially lethal as the symptomatic kind. When a symptomatic infarction occurs, prognosis
is better if the patient did not have angina preceding the infarction.

REFERENCES

1. G. J. Goldman and A. D. Pichard. The natural history of coronary artery disease: Does medical therapy improve the prognosis? *Prog. Cardiovasc. Dis.*, *25*:513 (1983).
2. W. B. Kannel, P. Sorlie, and P. M. McNamara. Prognosis after initial myocardial infarction: The Framingham Study. *Am. J. Cardiol.*, *44*:53 (1979).
3. W. B. Kannel and R. D. Abbott. Incidence and prognosis of unrecognized myocardial infarction: Based on 26 years follow-up in the Framingham Study. In *Silent Myocardial Ischemia* (W. Rutishauser and H. Roskamm, eds.), Springer–Verlag, Berlin, 1984, pp. 131–137.
4. W. B. Kannel and R. D. Abbott. Incidence and prognosis of unrecognized myocardial infarction. An update on the Framingham Study. *N. Engl. J. Med.*, *311*:1144 (1984).
5. J. H. Medalie and M. A. Goldbourt. Unrecognized myocardial infarction: Five-year incidence, mortality and risk factors. *Ann. Intern. Med.*, *84*:526 (1976).
6. R. W. Harper, G. Kennedy, R. W. DeSanctis, and A. M. Hutter, Jr. The incidence and pattern of angina prior to acute myocardial infarction: A study of 577 cases. *Am. Heart J.*, *97*: 178 (1979).
7. M. Matsuda, Y. Matsuda, H. Ogawa, K. Moritani, and R. Kusukawa. Angina pectoris before and during acute myocardial infarction: Relation to degree of physical activity. *Am. J. Cardiol.*, *55*:1255 (1985).
8. J. Midwall, J. Ambrose, A. Pichard, Z. Abedin, and M. V. Herman. Angina pectoris before and after myocardial infarction: angiographic correlations. *Chest*, *81*:681 (1982).
9. Y. Matsuda, H. Ogawa, K. Moritani, M. Matsuda, H. Naito, M. Matsuzaki, Y. Ikee, and R. Kusukawa. Effects of the presence or absence of preceding angina pectoris on left ventricular function after acute myocardial infarction. *Am. Heart J.*, *108*: 955 (1984).
10. A. Cortina, J. A. Ambrose, J. Prieto-Granada, C. Moris, E. Simarro, J. Holt, and V. Fuster. Left ventricular function after myocardial infarction: Clinical and angiographic correlations. *J. Am. Coll. Cardiol.*, *5*:619 (1985).

V
MANAGEMENT OF PATIENTS WITH ASYMPTOMATIC CORONARY ARTERY DISEASE

15
Medical Treatment of Asymptomatic Coronary Artery Disease

Perhaps no single area concerning asymptomatic coronary artery disease is as controversial as management [1]. Although "hard-data" are sparse, certain recommendations can be offered on the basis of the prognostic information provided in the preceding section.

I. MANAGEMENT OF PERSONS WHO ARE TOTALLY ASYMPTOMATIC

Because the prognosis in persons in this category is generally favorable, the simplest approach is to (1) modify risk factors when they are present and (2) reduce physical activities so that myocardial ischemia does not develop. The latter is to ward off possible damage to the patient with a defective angina warning system [2] during strenuous exertion. It is those patients who demonstrate extensive ischemia that merit special concern [3]. These individuals are more likely to have multivessel disease with its correspondingly worse prognosis. As opposed to asymptomatic persons with single-vessel disease who may be in a "presymptomatic" stage and go on to angina or nonfatal infarction, asymptomatic individuals with triple-vessel or left main disease appear to be at higher risk for sudden death or massive infarctions. Every effort should be made to treat these patients with antiischemic agents, thereby improving exercise tolerance by prolonging the time at which ischemia develops. Improvement in ischemic zones could be documented in one of several ways. For example, in a pilot study from our laboratory [4], we treated eleven patients with silent myocardial ischemia (some of whom had prior infarctions) with beta-blockers and evaluated exercise ECGs and radionuclide ventriculograms before and after administration of the drugs. The beneficial results are depicted in Table 1. Whether prognosis is improved in these patients cannot be proven at present, but it is an attractive hypothesis because of a postulated link between catecholamine-induced hypokalemia and ventricular arrhythmias in coronary patients. Noncardioselective beta-blockers can reverse this type of hypokalemia [5, 6] and may be especially useful in persons with extensive disease and defective angina warning systems who are prone to develop serious arrhythmias and sudden death during exertion.

Another "medical" approach in selected asymptomatic patients is coronary angioplasty. This relatively new procedure has received widespread acceptance because of its low complication rate and high success rate [7]. It is especially well suited for asymptomatic patients with very severe proximal lesions of the left anterior descending coronary artery.

Psychological counseling is also important in these patients since the implications of a potentially lethal but silent disease can

Table 1 Treatment of Silent Myocardial Ischemia with Beta-Adrenergic Blockage (BAB)

	Pre-BAB	Post-BAB	p Value
Time to exercise-induced ST depression	207 sec ± 75	348 sec ± 89	p < 0.05
Maximum ST depression	1.41 mm ± 0.15	0.81 ± 0.20	p < 0.05
Change in regional exercise ejection fraction	−0.06 ± 0.01	−0.01 ± 0.01	p < 0.01

by anxiety-provoking and detrimental to the patient's emotional well-being [8]. This is discussed further in the following section on postinfarction patients.

II. MANAGEMENT OF PATIENTS WHO ARE ASYMPTOMATIC FOLLOWING A MYOCARDIAL INFARCTION

There is a greater consensus concerning treatment of these patients. Those who are skeptical of treating totally asymptomatic persons would treat postinfraction patients with silent ischemia [9]. Even in patients who do *not* have a positive stress test before discharge from the hospital, treatment with beta-blockers is recommended. to reduce short-term mortality and reinfarction [10]. In my opinion, certainly all patients with evidence of myocardial ischemia postinfarction should receive this treatment. The effectiveness is confirmed in Table 1. If beta-blockers are contraindicated, then calcium antagonists should be used.

As discussed previously in Chapter 11, many physicians regard continuing evidence of ischemia as grounds for cardiac catheterization. Depending on the severity of the angiographic findings, some of these patients will be candidates for more aggressive medical management, coronary angioplasty, or coronary bypass surgery. Comparisons of medical versus surgical management (as in the CASS survey) will be discussed in the next chapter.

Psychological reactions in these patients are also important, since many assume that once they have recovered from the acute infarction and are asymptomatic, they have little to worry about. When this assumption is corrected, the level of anxiety is raised [8]. However, in a study of 15 patients with asymptomatic coronary artery disease, most of whom had prior infarctions, we found that most patients felt their physicians had been supportive in explaining the problems to them. Because of trust in their physicians, patients often changed their lifestyles markedly in regard to exercise and diet. All agreed that public awareness of this disorder was unfortunately almost non-existent.

III. MANAGEMENT OF PATIENTS WITH EPISODES OF BOTH SYMPTOMATIC AND ASYMPTOMATIC MYOCARDIAL ISCHEMIA

This group of patients are the most numerous group that practitioners will encounter. In the past, there has been a tendency to discount the importance of the asymptomatic episodes and to treat "symptoms." With the report of several groups [11–15] that asymptomatic episodes often greatly outnumber symptomatic episodes (as determined by Holter monitoring), there is a growing trend toward considering the asymptomatic episodes of equal importance. If this trend continues — and there is every reason to expect that it will — a new approach to the treatment of myocardial ischemia will be employed [16]. In this approach, the use of drugs, angioplasty, and surgery will be to reduce the *total* number of ischemic episodes and not merely the symptomatic ones.

Choice of medications in these patients (as in all coronary patients) depends on the *type* of ischemia that is present, i.e., whether it is due to increased work of the heart or to a vasospastic component or both. In the former case, myocardial oxygen requirements are raised, usually because of increases in heart rate and blood pressure, two of the major factors regulating myocardial oxygen consumption (Table 2). For these episodes, "prophylactic" beta-blockers would appear to be reasonable agents.

However, many of the episodes do *not* appear to be associated with increased work of the heart. For example, Schang and Pepine (see Figure 6 in Chapter 8) [10] and more recently Cecchi et al. (Figure 1) [11] reported that the ratio of asymptomatic episodes

Table 2   Major Determinants of Myocardial Oxygen Consumption

1. Heart rate
2. Intramyocardial tension (a function of blood pressure and ventricular volume)
3. Myocardial contractility

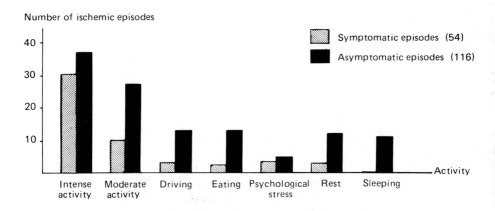

Figure 1   Activity at the onset of ischemic attacks. Intense physical activity-jogging, playing tennis, bicycling, walking upstairs and sexual activity. Moderate physical activity-slow walking, light housework and light hand labor. (From A. C. Cecchi, E. V. Dovellini, F. Marchi, P. Pucci, C. M. Santoro, and P. F. Fazzini. *J. Am. Coll. Cardiol., 1*:934, 1983.)

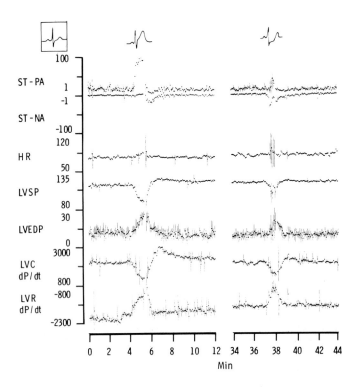

Figure 2   Computer plot of two asymptomatic ischemic episodes in the same patient. The averaged values of each derived variable are plotted with their standard deviation against time. The variables (top to bottom) were ST segment positive (PA) and negative areas (NA), heart rate (HR), left ventricular systolic (LVSP) and end-diastolic pressures (LVEDP) and left ventricular peak contraction (LVC) and relaxation (LVR) dP/dt. In the episode on the left, transient ST segment elevation (increase in ST segment positive area) was accompanied by an increase in left ventricular end-diastolic pressure, and decreases in both contraction and relaxation peak dP/dt. Similar impairment of left ventricular function accompanied the asymptomatic episode of ST segment depression (increase in ST segment negative area) in the same electrocardiographic lead shown on the right. A vasospastic component is suggested by the lack of increase in the variables controlling myocardial oxygen demand (such as HR or LVSP) before either episode. (From S. Chierchia, M. Lazzari, B. Freedman, C. Brunelli, and A. Maseri. *J. Am. Coll. Cardiol.*, *1*:924, 1983).

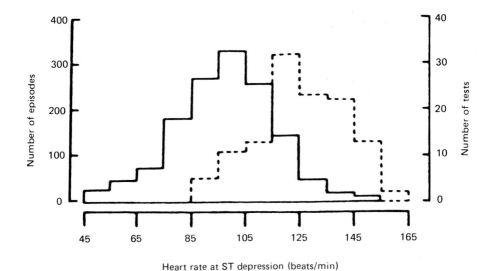

Figure 3   Distribution of heart rates at onset of ST depression during ambulatory monitoring (———) and during exercise testing (— — — —). (From J. E. Deanfield, A. P. Selwyn, S. Krikler, and M. Morgan. *Lancet, 2:*753, 1983.)

recorded on Holter monitoring was greatest during nonstrenuous activities. This suggests a vasospastic mechanism. Further evidence is provided by the lack of increased heart rate or blood pressure preceding many episodes, as in the example in Figure 2, from the study of Chierchi et al. [12]. Deanfield et al. [13, 14] also showed that in their patients the heart rate at the onset of ST segment depression was significantly lower after unprovoked ischemia than after exercise (Figure 3). Peak heart rates showed the same trend. During silent myocardial ischemia due to mental stress, heart rate was also less than during exercise-induced ischemia [17]. For episodes of silent ischemia not associated with increased work of the heart, nitrates or calcium antagonists would provide the best approach to therapy. Schang and Pepine [11] were able to significantly reduce the frequency of asymptomatic episodes using hourly nitroglycerin tablets (3.7 ± 0.02 episodes per monitoring period to 0.6 ± 0.02). Johnson et al. [18] reduced total ischemic episodes with verapamil in Prinzmetal's angina; Oakley et al. [19] did the same with propranolol and nifedipine in patients with typical angina.

IV. MANAGEMENT OF SILENT MYOCARDIAL INFARCTION

Recognition of these events invariably occurs too late for the usual treatment accorded patients with infarctions. However, patients at times may present with the *complications* of a silent infarction and require appropriate management. An example is the patient in pulmonary edema reported by Raper et al. [20].

V. CONCLUSIONS

Medical management of silent myocardial ischemia involves modification of risk factors, use of drugs and, in appropriate patients, angioplasty. Although beta-blockade appears efficacious during exertion, many of the ischemic episodes appear to have a vasospastic component, suggesting that calcium antagonists may also be of value.

REFERENCES

1. P. F. Cohn, E. J. Brown, Jr., and J. K. Cohn. Detection and management of coronary artery disease in the asymptomatic population. *Am. Heart J., 108*:1064 (1984).
2. P. F. Cohn. Silent myocardial ischemia in patients with a defective anginal warning system. *Am. J. Cardiol., 45*:697 (1980).
3. P. F. Cohn. When is concern about silent myocardial ischemia justified? *Ann. Int. Med., 100*:597 (1984).
4. P. F. Cohn and E. J. Brown. Can silent myocardial ischemia during exercise be treated effectively with beta-adrenergic blocking agents? (Abstr.) *Clin. Res., 33*:177A (1985).
5. M. J. Brown, D. C. Brown, and M. B. Murphy. Hypokalemia from $beta_2$-receptor stimulation by circulating epinephrine. *N. Engl. J. Med., 309*:1414 (1983).
6. H. H. Vincent, F. Boomsma, A. J. Man in't Veld, F. H. M. Derkx, G. J. Wenting, and M. A. D. H. Schalekamp. Effects of selective and nonselective β-agonists on plasma potassium and norepinephrine. *J. Cardiovasc. Pharmacol., 6*:107 (1984).
7. M. J. Cowley and P. C. Block. Percutaneous transluminal coronary angioplasty. *Mod. Concepts Cardiovasc. Dis., 50*: 25 (1981).
8. J. K. Cohn and P. F. Cohn. Patient reactions to the diagnosis of asymptomatic coronary artery disease: Implications for the

primary physician and consultant cardiologist. *J. Am. Coll. Cardiol.*, *1*:956 (1983).

9. R. F. Leighton and T. D. Fraker, Jr. Silent myocardial ischemia: Concern is justified for the patient with known coronary artery disease. *Ann. Intern. Med.*, *100*:599 (1984).
10. G. S. May, C. D. Kurberg, K. A. Eberlein, and B. J. Geraci. Secondary prevention after myocardial infarction: A review of short-term acute phase trials. *Prog. Cardiovasc. Dis.*, *25*: 335 (1983).
11. J. J. Schang, Jr., and C. J. Pepine. Transient asymptomatic ST-segment depression during daily activity. *Am. J. Cardiol.*, *39*:396 (1977).
12. A. C. Cecchi, E. V. Dovellini, F. Marchi, P. Pucci, C. M. Santoro, and P. F. Fazzini. Silent myocardial ischemia during ambulatory electrocardiographic monitoring in patients with effort angina. *J. Am. Coll. Cardiol.*, *1*:934 (1983).
13. S. Chierchia, M. Lazzari, B. Freedman, C. Brunelli, and A. Maseri. Impairment of myocardial perfusion and function during painless myocardial ischemia. *J. Am. Coll. Cardiol.*, *1*:924 (1983).
14. J. E. Deanfield, A. P. Selwyn, S. Chierchia, A. Maseri, P. Ribeiro, S. Krikler, and M. Morgan. Myocardial ischemia during daily life in patients with stable angina: Its relation to symptoms and heart rate changes. *Lancet*, *2*:753 (1983).
15. J. E. Deanfield, M. Shea, P. Ribiero, C. M. deLandsheere, R. A. Wilson, P. Horlock, and A. P. Selwyn. Transient ST segment depression as a marker of myocardial ischemia during daily life: A physiological validation in patients with angina and coronary disease. *Am. J. Cardiol.*, *54*:1195 (1984).
16. P. F. Cohn. Time for a new approach to the management of patients with both symptomatic and asymptomatic episodes of myocardial ischemia. *Am. J. Cardiol.*, *54*:1357 (1984).
17. J. E. Deanfield, M. Kensett, R. A. Wilson, M. Shea, P. Horlock, C. M. deLandsheere, and A. P. Selwyn. Silent myocardial ischemia due to mental stress. *Lancet*, *2*:1001 (1984).
18. S. M. Johnson, D. R. Mauritson, J. T. Willerson, and L. D. Hillis. A controlled trial of verapamil for Prinzmetal's variant angina. *N. Engl. J. Med.*, *304*:862 (1981).
19. G. D. G. Oakley, K. M. Fox, H. J. Dargie, and A. P. Selwyn. Objective assessment of therapy in severe angina. *Br. Med. J.*, *1*:1540 (1979).

20. A. J. Raper, A. Hastillo, and W. J. Paulsen. The syndrome of sudden severe painless myocardial ischemia. *Am. Heart J., 107*: 813 (1984).

16

Surgical Treatment of Asymptomatic Coronary Artery Disease

Some investigators are adamantly against surgery in asymptomatic patients in general; others are in favor of it in very limited circumstances; yet others take a broader view. Unfortunately, many of the surgical series have no medical controls and, therefore, do not provide enough "light," merely "heat." Furthermore, in most instances, there is no documentation that these asymptomatic patients still demonstrate myocardial ischemia preoperatively.

Table 1   Surgical Therapy in Asymptomatic Patients with
Coronary Artery Disease[a] (Nonrandomized Studies)

Reporting Institution	No. of Patients	Perioperative Mortality	Mean Follow-up (mo)	Late Mortality
Cleveland Clinic	17	0	75	0
University of Washington	392	15(3.8%)	65	NA
Peter Bent Brigham	20	0	34	1(5%)
Montreal Heart Institute	55	0	69	4(7.3%)

[a]All studies include patients with prior myocardial infarction. University of
Washington, Peter Bent Brigham and Montreal Heart Institute studies also in-
clude patients with mild symptoms.
NA = not available.

Because surgical patients who are totally asymptomatic are small in
number, they are usually combined in follow-up reports with
patients who are asymptomatic following a myocardial infarction.
In addition, at the present time, there is no specific surgical data on
patients with angina who have frequent asymptomatic episodes.
For these reasons, I have not used the same subheadings as in other
chapters but rather discuss the findings in terms of nonrandomized
versus randomized studies. The latter are more numerous and will
be discussed first.

I. NONRANDOMIZED STUDIES

Coronary bypass surgery in small numbers of asymptomatic patients
has been performed at several hospitals (Table 1). Usually these
patients are reported as part of a mixed series that includes asymptomatic and mildly symptomatic patients. The results involving the
asymptomatic patients must then be dissected out from the main
body of data. The study from the Seattle Heart Watch conducted
by the University of Washington School of Medicine [1] is one such

study. In this series, 114 patients were asymptomatic and 505 patients were mildly symptomatic. Prognosis was compared in medically and surgically treated patients. Even though the study was nonrandomized, it provides important data because the medically and surgically treated patients had similar baseline variables. The surgically treated patients had a lower mortality (via life-table analyses) then their medical counterparts, with the largest difference in survival seen in patients with triple-vessel disease and ejection fractions between 31 and 50% (Figure 1). This is the only controlled study of this type that suggests a beneficial effect of surgery on mortality in asymptomatic patients. Because prognosis in patients with normal ejection fractions and mild or no symptoms appeared excellent, the authors did not feel anything but an enormous sample size would be sufficient to test the hypothesis that surgical therapy improves survival in that type of patient. Furthermore, there were too few asymptomatic patients with left main lesions for the authors to make any definite statements about treatment for that lesion, but they did feel that on the basis of their study, they would recommend surgery in patients with triple-vessel disease and moderate impairment of left ventricular function.

In addition to the retrospective "matched" study indicated above, there have also been several reports of surgical series without attempts to have control groups. Thus, Grondin et al. [2], at the Montreal Heart Institute, reported on 55 patients, 19 of whom were totally asymptomatic. Most patients had multivessel disease. There were four late deaths and seven late infarctions in the 69-month follow-up period, and despite the zero perioperative mortality, the authors questioned the value of this type of prophylactic surgery. Thurer et al. [3] operated on 17 patients at the Cleveland Clinic who were asymptomatic after an infarction. Sixteen of the seventeen remained asymptomatic. The Peter Bent Brigham Hospital [4] experience was similar (Table 2). Twenty patients were studied, 14 of whom were totally asymptomatic. Six of these had sustained a prior myocardial infarction. This series was unique in that 16 patients had preoperative exercise tests, of which 14 demonstrated silent ischemia. The only death in this series occurred five years after surgery. There were 12 patients with both preoperative and postoperative exercise tests; in eight the test became completely normal, while in the other four, less of an ischemic

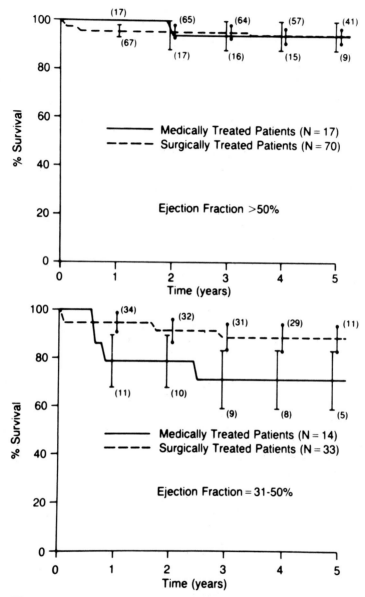

Figure 1 Actuarial survival curves comparing medically and surgically treated patients with three-vessel disease subgrouped according to ejection fraction. (From K. E. Hammermeister, T. A. DeRouen, and H. T. Dodge. *Circulation, 62*:98, 1980.)

Table 2   Clinical Data on Patients with Minimal or no Angina
Pectoris who Underwent CABG Surgery

Pt. no.	Age	MI	Angina pectoris	ETT Preop	ETT Postop	Diseased vessels (no.)	Grafts (no.)	Follow-up (mos)
1	49	+	−	0	0	2	2	80
2	54	−	−	+	−	LM	1	63
3	47	+	−	−	−	3	2	62(1)
4	58	+	−	0	0	3	5	53
5	53	+	−	+	−	3	3	42
6	35	+	−	+	−	2	3	39
7	42	−	=	+	−	3	3	36
8	49	+	−	0	−	2	1	30
9	36	−	−	+	+	2	2	30
10	39	+	−	+	−	2	2	29
11	63	+	=	+	−	3	3	28
12	37	−	=	+	0	3	5	23
13	44	−	−	+	0	3	2	23
14	62	−	−	+	+	3	3	22
15	60	+	=	+	+	LM	3	22
16	43	+	=	−	0	2	3	21
17	55	−	=	+	−	LM	3	21
18	55	+	−	0	−	3	3	21
19	53	−	−	+	+	1	2	20
20	50	−	−	+	−	LM	2	19

CABG = coronary artery bypass surgery; ETT = exercise tolerance test; + =
positive or present; − = negative or absent; = = mild; 0 = not done; D = late
death; LM = left main coronary; MI = prior myocardial infarction.
(From J. Wynne, L. H. Cohn, J. J. Collins, Jr., and P. F. Cohn. *Circulation*,
58(Suppl I):I-92, 1978.)

A.

PREOPERATIVE

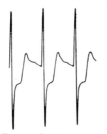

5 -mm ST Depression
Heart Rate: 145 beats/min
Duration of Exercise: 4.5 min

POSTOPERATIVE

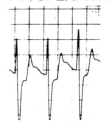

2-mm ST Depression
Heart Rate: 150 beats/min
Duration of Exercise: 10.5 min

B.

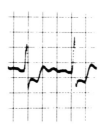

Positive 3-mm ST Depression
Heart Rate: 108 beats/min
Duration of Exercise: 7 min

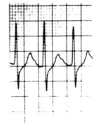

Negative
Heart Rate: 165 beats/min
Duration of Exercise: 10 min

Figure 2   Representative leads (V_4) from preoperative (left) and postoperative (right) exercise tolerance tests in two patients demonstrating improvement after surgery. (A) Improvement in degree of ST segment depression, and duration of exercise. (B) Normalization of ST segment response to exercise, and improvement in duration of exercise. (From J. Wynne, L. H. Cohn, J. J. Collins, Jr., and P. F. Cohn. *Circulation*, *58*(Suppl 1):1-92, 1978.)

response was observed compared to the preoperative test. Examples of these exercise tests are depicted in Figure 2. Fitzgibbon et al. [5] reported on a series of 723 consecutive patients operated on between 1971–1979. The authors separated the 118 patients who had no angina three years prior to the study from the 605 who had angina. No important differences in survival between the patients was noted.

II. RANDOMIZED STUDIES

The multicenter Coronary Artery Surgery Study (CASS) [6] has provided additional data against surgical intervention. Unlike the Seattle report, this was a randomized study, but one with certain qualifying features. First, most patients had sustained myocardial infarctions. Second, they all had undergone coronary arteriography prior to randomization. Third, patients with left main lesions or ejection fractions less than 0.35 were excluded. Fourth, although only patients with no angina or mild angina (Class I and II NYHA) were included, many patients required medication to attain this pain-free or mild-pain classification. From the original 16,626 patients who underwent coronary arteriography at 15 sites from 1974 to 1979, 780 patients with stable ischemic heart disease were randomized to medical or surgical therapy; 390 patients were in each group (Figure 3). There were no statistically significant differences in survival in patients receiving medical versus surgical therapy. This applied not only to the entire cohort, but also the various subgroups based on extent of vessel disease or left ventricular ejection fraction. There was a trend toward better surgical results in the <0.50 ejection fraction group, but the numbers of patients with one- and two-vessel disease and low ejection fractions were so small as to make statistics meaningless. Numbers were larger in the triple-vessel-disease subgroup and the annual mortality with medical treatment was twice that of the surgical group (4% vs. 2%). However, the number of patients was again not large enough to reach statistical significance at five years (Figure 4) although this did occur at seven years (5.2% vs. 1.7%, $p < 0.01$) [7]. Additional criticism of the CASS experience has dealt with the fact that the final number of patients (780) may not truly reflect prognosis in the other 93.5% of the patients who were not randomized. It is important to note that no data on ischemia induced by stress testing were provided with the survival data. As discussed earlier in

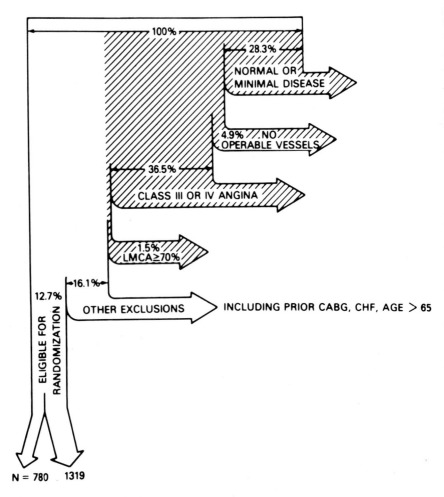

Figure 3   Allocation of 16,626 patients in CASS registry at randomizing sites. Reasons for exclusion of patients from study. Width is proportional to the number of patients in each category. LMCA = left main coronary artery; CABG = coronary artery bypass graft; CHF = congestive heart failure. (From CASS Principal Investigators and their Associates. *Circulation, 68*:939, 1983.)

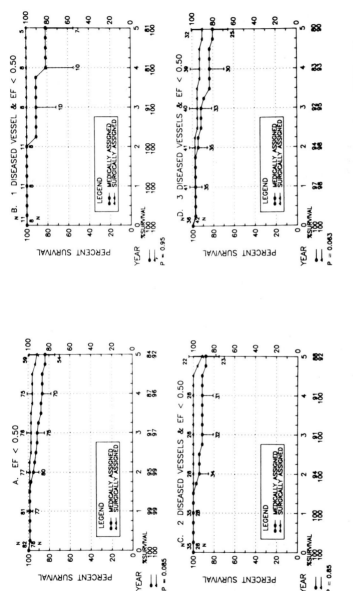

Figure 4 Five-year cumulative survival rates for patients with ejection fractions (EF) of less than 0.50 (A) and patients with ejection fractions of less than 0.50 and single- (B), double- (C) and triple- (D) vessel disease. Numbers of patients followed each year are on the survival curves. (From CASS Principal Investigators and their Associates. *Circulation*, 68:939, 1983.)

Chapter 12, the existence of high-risk patients within the three-vessel disease subgroup can be verified only when additional tests beside the angiogram are performed. Therefore, we do not know if the low mortality in the medically treated group reflects treatment of these high-risk patients. Furthermore, the study does not make clear what level of medication was necessary to reach the asymptomatic state. Nevertheless, it must be remembered that this is not a natural history study of no-treatment versus treatment, but rather medical versus surgical treatment. In that context, it does provide comparative survival figures for medically and surgically treated patients in the 1970s.

A smaller randomized trial of medical versus surgical management was carried out at Green Lane Hospital in New Zealand [8]. One hundred patients who were asymptomatic after a myocardial infarction were followed for a mean period of four and a half years. Annual mortality was 2% in both groups. These patients had at least two infarcts and had to survive at least two months postinfarction to be included in the randomization process. The patients — most with extensive coronary artery disease — again had a surprisingly low annual mortality and most were not on beta-blocking agents. This again makes it difficult for surgical survival to be "better." Furthermore, of the four surgical deaths, one was from noncardiac causes and one died while awaiting surgery. This study has been criticized because of the two-month lag before randomization began; it is in this period that most of the medical deaths occur.

III. CONCLUSIONS

After reviewing this data, what is one to conclude? Should surgery be withheld from asymptomatic patients, as some argue [9]? Or is it indicated in selected instances such as patients with left main or triple-vessel disease, and left ventricular dysfunction, as others maintain [10]? In my view, it is the latter opinion that provides the best guidelines at present. Patients with less extensive disease can be managed with medical therapy and, at times, with angioplasty.

Although survival figures are obviously a "hard" end-point, evaluation of patients after surgery must also consider whether ischemia has been relieved. This is difficult to evaluate subjectively but it can be done with objective tests of myocardial function such as exercise tests or ambulatory monitoring. The latter represents a

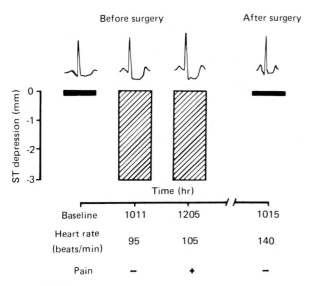

Figure 5   Ambulatory electrocardiograms in a patient showing two episodes of ST segment depression, one painful (+) and one painless (−), before coronary surgery. After surgery no episode of ST depression was recorded even at higher heart rates. (From P. Ribeiro, M. Shea, J. E. Deanfield, C. M. Oakley, R. Sapsford, T. Jones, R. Walesby and A. P. Selwyn. *Br. Heart J.*, *52*:502, 1984.)

new approach that may be especially useful in evaluating patients with both symptomatic and asymptomatic episodes (Figure 5) [11]. As with exercise testing, residual ischemic episodes without pain may be demonstrated. Whether they will influence long-term prognosis remains to be seen.

REFERENCES

1. K. E. Hammermeister, T. A. DeRouen, and H. T. Dodge. Effect of coronary surgery on survival in asymptomatic and minimally symptomatic patients. *Circulation*, *62*:98 (1980).
2. C. M. Grondin, J. G. Kretz, P. Vouhe, J. F. Tubau, L. Compeau, and M. G. Bourassa. Prophylactic coronary artery grafting in patients with few or no symptoms. *Ann. Thorac. Surg.*, *28*: 113 (1978).

3. R. L. Thurer, B. W. Lytle, D. M. Cosgrove, and F. D. Loop.
    Asymptomatic coronary artery disease managed by myocardial
    revascularization: Results at 5 years. *Circulation, 61*(Suppl
    1):1–14 (1976).
4. J. Wynne, L. H. Cohn, J. J. Collins, Jr., and P. F. Cohn. Myo-
    cardial revascularization in patients with multivessel coronary
    artery disease and minimal angina pectoris. *Circulation, 58*
    (Suppl I):I–92 (1978).
5. G. M. FitzGibbon, J. R. Burton, and W. J. Keon. Aortocoronary
    bypass surgery in "asymptomatic" patients with coronary
    artery disease. In *Silent Myocardial Ischemia* (W. Rutishauser
    and H. Roskamm, eds.), Springer–Verlag, Berlin, 1984, pp.
    180–193.
6. CASS Principal Investigators and their Associates. Coronary
    Artery Surgery Study (CASS): A randomized trial of coronary
    artery bypass surgery: Survival data. *Circulation, 68*:939
    (1983).
7. E. Passamani, K. B. Davis, M. J. Gillespie, T. Killip, and the
    CAS Principal Investigators and their associates. A randomized
    trial of coronary artery bypass usrgery. Survival of patients
    with a low ejection fraction. *N. Engl. J. Med., 312*:1665 (1985).
8. R. M. Norris, T. M. Agnes, P. W. T. Brandt, K. J. Graham, D.
    G. Jill, A. R. Kerr, J. B. Lowe, A. H. G. Roche, R. M. L.
    Whitlock, and B. G. Barrett-Boyes. Coronary surgery after a
    recurrent myocardial infarction: Progress of a trial comparing
    surgical with nonsurgical management for asymptomatic
    patients with advanced coronary disease. *Circulation, 63*:
    785 (1981).
9. A. Selzer and K. Cohn. Asymptomatic coronary artery disease
    and coronary bypass surgery. *Am. J. Cardiol., 39*:614 (1977).
10. K. M. Kent, D. R. Rosing, C. J. Ewels, L. Kipson, R. Bonow,
    and S. E. Epstein. Prognosis of asymptomatic or mildly
    symptomatic patients with coronary artery disease. *Am. J.
    Cardiol., 49*:1823 (1982).
11. P. Ribeiro, M. Shea, J. E. Deanfield, C. M. Oakley, R. Sapsford,
    T. Jones, R. Walesby, and A. P. Selwyn. Different mechanisms
    for the relief of angina after coronary bypass surgery: Physio-
    logical versus anatomical assessment. *Br. Heart J., 52*:502
    (1984).

VI
FUTURE DIRECTIONS

17
Silent Myocardial Ischemia and Silent Myocardial Infarction
What issues remain to be resolved?

   I. Silent Myocardial Ischemia
  II. Silent Myocardial Infarction
     References

Despite the numerous studies of asymptomatic coronary artery disease described in the preceding pages, it is clear that there are still more unresolved issues than there are resolved issues.

I. SILENT MYOCARDIAL ISCHEMIA

To begin with, present and future lines of investigation must include more emphasis on the pathophysiologic mechanisms of silent myocardial ischemia. Can the work of Droste and Roskamm [1] on experimental pain thresholds be confirmed? Is there indeed an alteration in the somatic pain mechanisms in some of these individuals? If so, what is the relationship to cardiac pain, that elusive entity that has proven so difficult to define? If there is an alteration in somatic or cardiac pain perception, is this alteration found only in individuals with Type 1 or Type 2 silent ischemia? Do anginal patients with episodes of silent ischemia (Type 3 patients) have a different pathophysiologic mechanism, i.e., less myocardium at jeopardy? The studies from Maseri's laboratory [2] would seem to suggest this is the operative mechanism in this type of patient, but better techniques to quantitate the amount of ischemic myocardium — during both symptomatic and asymptomatic episodes — will be necessary for this hypothesis to be confirmed. In addition, the widespread use of angioplasty now offers a safe way of "inducing" transient ischemia in an acceptable manner and should lead to more data for comparisons of the symptomatic versus the asymptomatic episode.

Estimates of the prevalence of the various types of silent myocardial ischemia are more of a "guestimate" at present. While it will be difficult logistically and financially for one center in the United States to duplicate Erikssen's Norwegian study [3], it would certainly be interesting to see the results of this kind of diagnostic approach in Type 1 persons in a multicentered study in the United States. The cost of this kind of study might still argue against its feasibility, as would the question of confirmatory coronary angiography. It would probably be much simpler to obtain hard data on the prevalence of silent ischemia in asymptomatic *postinfarction* patients (Type 2). The frequency of exercise testing (and Holter monitor studies) in this subgroup make it a fertile source of information. Similarly, Holter monitoring in angina patients should provide reliable figures on the prevalence of Type 3 silent ischemia.

Studies that establish the prevalence of the three types of silent myocardial ischemia can also be used to obtain more natural history data, as Erikssen has done in his investigations [4]. Unfortunately, there are no similar *prospective* studies in Types 2 and 3. Are Holter monitors reliable enough to provide such data? What of the next generation of these devices? Will they be more suitable for ST segment recording? Such studies are essential for making intelligent management decisions. But management decisions will require more than natural history data. Here is where the circulatory dynamics of the ischemic episodes come into play. Is there a vasospastic component and, therefore, are nitrates and calcium antagonists better suited for this syndrome than beta-adrenergic blocking agents? Should the latter be used only in exertion-induced episodes? Finally, what happens to the subgroup of patients with left main and/or three-vessel disease? Are they truly as susceptible to sudden death and massive infarcts as suggested by the Norwegian data, or is their course more benign and similar to the asymptomatic individual with one-vessel disease? More data are needed.

II. SILENT MYOCARDIAL INFARCTION

We have made important strides in documenting the prevalence of silent myocardial infarction; the Framingham Study [5] is a good example of this kind of prospective investigation. Again, as in silent myocardial ischemia, we are not sure why nondiabetic individuals do not experience pain with their infarcts. Even though this is "softer" data (because physicians do not observe the infarct as we do the transient episodes of silent ischemia), there is still much that can be learned about these patients. Are they also experiencing episodes of silent ischemia? What is the incidence of recurrent silent infarctions? With widespread Holter monitoring, we should document many more of these infarctions and their arrhythmic complications as they occur, which leads us to the last and perhaps most important issue. What is the relationship of silent ischemia and infarction to sudden cardiac death? Some evidence from Erikssen's study [4] supports this link, but more data are necessary. There are many aspects of sudden cardiac death that remain to be unraveled, but one aspect of this syndrome is particularly fascinating. Are these individuals experiencing silent ischemia prior to their demise? Certainly the few anecdotal reports from Sharma et al. [6] and others suggest that this is so. To take survivors of cardiac death and systematically test them for silent ischemia requires a concerted effort from several centers and by definition, we can only investigate survivors. Is this somehow a skewered population? This is one question we may never be able to answer.

REFERENCES

1. C. Droste and H. Roskamm. Experimental pain measurements in patients with asymptomatic myocardial ischemia. *J. Am. Coll. Cardiol.*, *1*:940 (1983).
2. S. Chierchia, M. Lazzari, B. Freedman, C. Brunelli, and A. Maseri. Impairment of myocardial perfusion and function during painless myocardial ischemia. *J. Am. Coll. Cardiol.*, *1*: 924 (1983).
3. J. Erikssen, I. Enge, K. Forfang, and O. Storstein. False positive diagnostic test and coronary angiographic findings in 105 presumably healthy males. *Circulation*, *54*:371 (1976).
4. J. Erikssen and E. Thaulow. Follow-up of patients with asymptomatic myocardial ischemia. In *Silent Myocardial Ischemia* (W. Rutishauser and H. Roskamm, eds.), Springer–Verlag, Berlin, 1984, pp. 156–164.
5. W. B. Kannel and R. D. Abbott. Incidence and prognosis of unrecognized myocardial infarction: An update on the Framingham Study. *N. Engl. J. Med.*, *311*:1144 (1984).
6. B. Sharma, G. Francis, M. Hodges, and R. Asinger. Demonstration of exercise-induced ischemia without angina in patients who recover from out-of-hospital ventricular fibrillation (abstr). *Am. J. Cardiol.*, *47*:445 (1981).

Index

A

Ambulatory electrocardio-
graphic (Holter)
monitoring, 105-121,
206, 209
Angina pectoris
circulatory dynamics of,
42-46
pathophysiology of,
compared to silent myo-
cardial ischemia, 42-46

[Angina pectoris]
prognosis of, compared to
silent myocardial ischemia,
179-184
treatment of, compared to
silent myocardial ischemia,
206-209, 213-233
unstable, prognostic significance
of painless episodes, 184
Apoprotein B, as marker for
asymptomatic coronary
artery disease, 97

DATE DUE

AP 8 96			